Learning Disability and Inclusion Phobia

The social position of learning disabled people has shifted rapidly over the last twenty years, from long-stay institutions, first into community homes and day centres, and now to a currently emerging goal of 'ordinary lives' for individuals using person-centred support and personal budgets. These approaches promise to replace a century and a half of 'scientific' pathological models based on expert assessment, and of the accompanying segregated social administration which determined how and where people led their lives, and who they were.

This innovative volume explains how concepts of learning disability, intellectual disability and autism first came about, describes their more recent evolution in the formal disciplines of psychology, and shows the direct relevance of this historical knowledge to present and future policy, practice and research. Goodey argues that learning disability is not a historically stable category and different people are considered 'learning disabled' as it changes over time. Using psychological and anthropological theory, he identifies the deeper lying pathology as 'inclusion phobia', in which the tendency of human societies to establish an ingroup and to assign outgroups reaches an extreme point. Thus the disability we call 'intellectual' is a concept essential only to an era in which to be human is essentially to be deemed intelligent, autonomous and capable of rational choice.

Interweaving the author's historical scholarship with his practice-based experience in the field, *Learning Disability and Inclusion Phobia* challenges myths about the past as well as about present-day concepts, exposing both the historical continuities and the radical discontinuities in thinking about learning disability.

C. F. Goodey is Honorary Fellow at the Centre for Medical Humanities, University of Leicester, having previously held teaching and research posts elsewhere in the UK at Ruskin College, the Open University and University College London Institute of Education. He is also an independent consultant on learning disability services for local government and national organizations. He is the author of *A History of Intelligence and 'Intellectual Disability': The Shaping of Psychology in Early Modern Europe.*

Routledge Advances in the Medical Humanities

Learning Disability and Inclusion Phobia

Past, present, future

C. F. Goodey

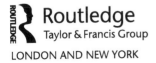

Routledge
Taylor & Francis Group

LONDON AND NEW YORK

First published 2016 by Routledge

2 Park Square, Milton Park, Abingdon, Oxfordshire OX14 4RN
711 Third Avenue, New York, NY 10017

Routledge is an imprint of the Taylor & Francis Group, an informa business

First issued in paperback 2017

British Library Cataloguing in Publication Data
A catalogue record for this book is available from the British Library

Library of Congress Cataloging-in-Publication Data
Goodey, C. F., author.
Learning disability and inclusion phobia : past, present, future /
C.F. Goodey.
p. ; cm. -- (Routledge advances in the medical humanities)
I. Title. II. Series: Routledge advances in the medical humanities.
[DNLM: 1. Intellectual Disability--history. 2. Community Integration--
history. 3. Education of Intellectually Disabled--history. 4. Intellectual
Disability--classification. 5. Social Marginalization--history. WM 11.1]
RC570
362.3--dc23
2015006452

ISBN: 978-0-415-82200-8 (hbk)
ISBN: 978-0-8153-5521-2 (pbk)

Typeset in Times New Roman
by Taylor & Francis Books

'Ahab had cherished a wild vindictiveness against the whale ... He at last came to identify with him, not only all his bodily woes, but all his intellectual and spiritual exasperations. ... As in his narrow-flowing monomania not one jot of Ahab's broad madness had been left behind; so in that broad madness not one jot of his great natural intellect had perished. ... Now in his heart Ahab had some glimpse of this, namely: all my means are sane, my motive and my object mad.'

Herman Melville, *Moby Dick*, Chapter 41.

Contents

A note on terminology

Several dozen different terms have been used even within the last century. This book employs three of them, occasionally even on the same page. If that seems complicated, it is not my fault. It reflects the real world. In many English-speaking countries the term 'learning disability' is restricted to specific issues such as dyslexia or attention deficit, as distinct from more general terms such as 'intellectual disability', or 'developmental disability' which overlaps with physical impairment. However, in the UK where this book was written, all three phrases are for everyday purposes synonymous. Learning disability is the one most often encountered, and is therefore used in the title, and throughout the book wherever the context is neutral.

As for 'intellectual disability', this tends to be confined to university departments. If I walked into a roomful of people and their families or even local practitioners in this country and asked 'Is this the intellectual disability session?' they would think I had stumbled into the wrong room. It is a particularly loaded label. It comes from cognitive psychology, a sub-discipline that has the temporary privilege of telling doctors, other professionals, the academy, and via them the rest of us, what intelligence is and therefore who we are. It encourages us to think that human beings, as a species, are defined exclusively by the capacity for information processing, logical reasoning and abstraction (categories whose basis in reality is, as we shall see, less certain than might be thought), rather than their capacity for, say, beauty, morals, or personal authenticity. I use the term 'intellectual disability' in places where those particular categories, or something like them, are being discussed.

Finally, when I have actual individuals in mind here, they are 'people with learning difficulties'. In the self-advocacy movement that is the term they most often want to be known by. If we are going to put people in boxes for the time being, it is the worst label apart from all the rest.

Acknowledgement

I am grateful to Ingrid Clark, Wilf Clark, Laura Davis, Linda Jordan and Pen Mendonça for supplying vital information, as have many people with learning difficulties and their families who over the years have contributed selflessly (and, it must seem to them, endlessly) to research, and/or who have directly pioneered change.

1   Introduction

What is learning disability? Any textbook will tell you. What is its place in the broader picture human beings have of each other? That is another question, and answers are needed. Doctors, psychologists, teachers, social workers, advocates, researchers, students, and last but first the people who currently carry the label, their families and friends: all of us need that bigger picture, and the longer view. We can understand practice, policy and research only in the context of time and place. Knowing where we all stand in that picture, where the idea of learning disability came from and where it may be going, is crucial to improving the lives of all of us. Without such an understanding, we operate in the dark.

Yet learning disability, as a concept, is usually spoken about as if what it is and what causes it can be taken for granted. Consider mental illness, by way of contrast. Currently its experts are in one of their periodic upheavals about what causes anomalies in the way people think and behave, and how to classify them. Genetic explanations, which have prevailed for a generation or more, are being challenged by a new wave of researchers who are once again doubting whether disorders such as neurosis, paranoia or bi-polar are something that is 'wrong' with people in a medical sense, rather than the result of what has happened to them over the course of their lives in society. Even so, those same experts would not dream of extending such doubts to Down's syndrome, Fragile X, autism or any such label, which seem without question to be innate and largely unalterable identities. But could these conditions, too, be just something that has happened to people over the course of their lives?

The answer is obviously No – as long as we just squint at the question through the tiny chink of our present moment in history. On the one hand, although the environment in its broad sense (from epigenetic factors at the early cellular stage through to life chances and education) may play some part in how people turn out, and can alter their basic abilities for better or worse just as it can for the rest of us, present forms of social organization seriously complicate life for some. On the other hand, although learning disability seems pre-set in individuals rather than something that just happens to them along the way, this does not exclude the possibility that it is something that has happened along the way to human cultures. Indeed, an exploration of the past confirms this. Go back far enough and there were no such people, as we shall see later – at least, not in the historical record. So how do we know 'they' were there at all?

If this book deconstructs the concept of learning disability, that is only one of its aims, and a secondary one at that. Just being sceptical and leaving things at that is no good to anyone. Its chief aim, with the demolition work done, is to *re*construct the concept as something else entirely, and to draw some consequences from this for the future in terms of policy and of people's lives. The past is relevant because reconstruction is the historian's core task, and because working with written archives can sometimes be as exact a science as working in a genetics lab. The book proposes that learning disability, as we see it today, is root and branch the product of a more general social phobia; and it proposes that this phobia, rather than learning disability as such, should be the object of our anxiety and the primary target of social and political action.

To define learning disability, we must first realize that under its various names it has been an idea on the move, with a starting point at a certain historical conjuncture and perhaps a future finishing point too. And even more than that, it is a shape-shifter. Definitions are transitory, and the people thus defined do not constitute some fixed and separate subspecies of humanity. Let two or three generations pass, and the individuals thus classified, along with their typical characteristics, will have changed. The underlying category, under whatever label (there have been literally dozens), is not cross-historical, and its modern version gradually disappears the further back we investigate. Not only is it a category on the move, it is just one in a broader pattern of other, equally shifting ways of people putting each other into boxes that may at first sight bear no relation to learning disability. The one thing they do have in common is that they are *status* categories. Learning disability is a passing phase in the broader history of how human beings represent themselves to themselves, and to their fellows – a history that undergoes constant and almost total transformation in the long term.

History helps us to isolate learning disability and intelligence and hold them up for more thorough inspection. It enables us to compare and contrast. I cannot promise the reader a cosy chronological ride from the caveman to the computer. The category and the people it describes are not hard facts of nature; they are current but temporary manifestations of a more resilient and long-term pathological condition observable at times across history in the extreme urge to exclude. Each chapter has some chronological sections, their purpose being to describe the changes in character of the population subjected to the phobia; but they only make sense when set alongside that pathological urge, whose unchanging structural presence is visible at most points in past or present. My illustrations from history and from the present are therefore often interwoven.

This may induce whiplash, but that is preferable to the alternative. Describing things only in the order in which they happened leads us astray. It encourages fables: for example that everything is getting better and better (as many biologists or medical professionals might see it), or that everything is getting worse and worse (as many social theorists might). Since my aim is to make good the fragility of the concept of learning disability by reconstructing it as the outcome of a more fundamental and long-lasting social pathology, most of the chapters conclude with history rather than starting with it. The fragility of our basic concepts is laid bare first, before building work can be undertaken on sounder historical foundations. Today needs yesterday to prepare for tomorrow.

I have brought together the two strands of my own background, in qualitative research around policy and advocacy on the one hand and in the academic history of ideas on the other. The first of these will be familiar territory for many readers, unlike the second, which is under-researched and which I broached in detail in an earlier book.[1] (Readers interested in the primary sources behind my historical summaries here should refer to the original.) That book left two questions hanging. First, if learning disability is not a permanent fact of nature, is the urge to exclude? The present book goes some but not all of the way to answering that unanswerable question. The second question concerns how the history of ideas interacts with social history. The only way we can understand either is with the aid of the other. It was important in the first book to make good the lack of research into the conceptual frameworks of the distant past and to compare those ideas with our own. Nevertheless, ideas do not make history unless real people, dominated by material social forces, are making it with them; these feature in the present book.

As for the future, the one thing a historical approach does tell us is that if things were so completely different in the past, they can be different again in the future. Even my own experience, that of a single lifetime, spans segregated long-stay institutions, their closure, the development of personalized support, the slow but tangible subordination of professional assessment to person-centred planning, the government's policy aim of 'ordinary lives' together with the backdoor reappearance of smaller-scale private institutions, and the introduction of and resistances to ordinary (mainstream) education. And even that one lifetime is no time at all in terms of the cultural changes we shall be looking at. Many of the people incarcerated in Western institutions even within the last century would not fit the learning disability category of today. Precursor categories such as the 'feeble-minded' contained unmarried mothers, their children, minor delinquents, misfits from chaotic families, waifs and strays, as well as some whom we would now label learning disabled.

And just as people who did, even then, fit our current category have emerged from their dungeons into daylight shared with everyone else, we are now creating a future in which there are new justifications for putting people away, by inventing categories, labels and institutions specifically for them. The autistic spectrum, non-existent two generations ago, and its associated system of special schools and private residential assessment and treatment centres, is an example. If the rapid turnover both in psychological categories and characteristics and in their corresponding social arrangements is visible to a living, still practising individual, how much more of a turnover can we expect from looking at the past or projecting into the future?

The point is to let this view of the link between past and future inform our thinking about the present. At various points in this book you may encounter some idea so bizarrely obsolete that you ask yourself, what has this got to do with me? Behind that thought is another, unexamined belief: that the only elements of the past that matter are the ones that look like the present. We have a huge investment in this assumption that present ideas are a modern improvement on primitive forebears. Why else work in the field? Nevertheless our present moment is ambiguous. On the one hand, there are oral historians like John Able, who tells us how he left his long-stay hospital for a place in the community,[2] or Mabel Cooper, who left the institution where for a quarter of a century she had slept in a locked sixty-bed dormitory with first-come-first-served clothes and toothbrushes to live an ordinary life in her own flat, shopping on her own, enjoying the company of children for the first time, and obtaining an honorary degree from the Open University.[3] Barb Goode, from a similar starting-point, wound up at the United Nations, delivering a speech on self-advocacy.[4] Yet while thousands of people like these have been liberated and found public attitudes more accepting than when they were first put away, we continue to hone the pre-natal diagnostic techniques whose aim is to prevent lives before they even begin.

The obvious question then arises: John, Mabel, Barb, do we want you around or don't we? However, this book does not engage in ethical debate. The questions start further back. Who and what is it we are actually talking about? Arguing about values will not get us far if we do not answer this question first. It is usually bypassed, not only by teachers and social workers whose knowledge of people with learning difficulties comes from direct involvement in their lives, but equally by doctors and psychologists, i.e. by those from whom we might expect the sort of knowledge that is precise, scientific, stable, and value-free. Consequently, at present, the person just *is* the label or category – no questions asked.

Plenty of critical questions about the general concept of disability, usually omitting learning disability, have been raised over the past generation. Readers familiar with this work will be familiar with some of the questions I raise here too, though I am not particularly concerned with theory of the linguistic variety (Foucault, Deleuze, etc.) that dominates such discussions. Doubts have been raised as to whether theory of this kind, particularly when applied to learning disability as distinct from mental illness, is actually Foucauldian at all.[5] Certainly its focus on language and its wariness of political action tend to inject a strong dose of pessimism about what can be achieved; and as someone whose motivation springs from close encounters with the professional opposition to person-centred service planning and desegregated schooling, I doubt whether discouragement is something I ever needed more of. Keen-eyed readers will no doubt detect a number of theoretical influences behind what I have written.

Chapter 2 states my starting hypothesis and does in fact discuss various ideas from psychiatry, anthropology and social psychology that might help to frame the rest of the discussion, while taking their limitations into account. Chapter 3 looks at the present fragility and past relativity of the concept of intelligence without which that of intellectual or learning disability could not exist. Chapter 4 examines the place of learning disability within the wider concept of difference, and the steps by which it came to occupy such a central position there. Chapter 5 discusses the role of biology and its relationship to the eugenic impulse in the modern construction of learning disability, noting how precarious is the very notion of a 'cause'. Chapter 6 identifies cognitive development as a characteristically modern notion which the concept of learning disability reinforces and vice-versa, and probes its religious as well as socio-economic roots. Chapter 7 places assessment and measurement in the wider context of general forms of discrimination, and traces the historical path by which these cross-historical forms became embedded within the very concept of learning disability. Chapter 8 analyses the very recent arrival of autism, contrasts it sharply with previous usages of the term, and investigates its future prospects as a replacement paradigm for learning disability. Chapter 9 lays out the wider framework of social anxieties and moral panics, historical and current, from which autism has emerged. Chapter 10 sets out the prospects for future work.

The more sharply defined our concept of learning disability, the more inevitable the segregating practices that go with it. Both concept and practice, from their Western origins, have taken over much of the rest of the world. Alongside Canada, the UK now has probably the most emancipatory adult policy directives around, which in pockets are being translated into practice. Yet the resistance runs deeper than can be imagined, and the examples I provide of that excluding urge from the UK show how prevalent its highly disturbing symptoms are here too. They must be all the clearer to readers in places where closed and segregated institutions are still the unquestioned norm. The urge to exclude on grounds of intelligence thrives in the modern world. Yet the practical case has been made and proven for including people in the same kinds of educational, employment and friendship groups as everyone else, demonstrating in practical detail how it can be and is (occasionally) done, without leaving anyone in the lurch.[6] We can close down all special schools, public segregated institutions and private care homes overnight, with the people in them becoming part of ordinary life. The problem is not doing it, but wanting it. This book says why.

Notes

1 C. Goodey (2011). *A History of Intelligence and 'Intellectual Disability': The Shaping of Psychology in Early Modern Europe*. Farnham: Ashgate.
2 J. Able (2008). *Cold Stone Floors and Carbolic Soap*. www.richmond.gov.uk/our_times_newsletter_march_09.pdf; and www.richmond.gov.uk/our_times_autumn_ 2008. pdf. Retrieved 14 April 2014.

3 M. Cooper (2012). *I'd Like to Know Why.* Ashill: Clover Press.
4 B. Goode (2011). *The Goode Life: Memoirs of Disability Rights Activist Barb Goode.* Vancouver: Spectrum.
5 M. Simpson (2013). *Modernity and the Appearance of Idiocy: Intellectual Disability as a Regime of Truth.* Lampeter: Mellen.
6 See for example J. O'Brien and C. Lyle O'Brien (2006). *Implementing Person Centred Planning: Voices of Experience.* Toronto: Inclusion Press; S. Taylor et al. (1987). *The Nonrestrictive Environment: On Community Integration of Persons with the Most Severe Disabilities.* Syracuse, NY: Human Policy Press. M. Falvey et al. (1997). *All My Life's a Circle. Using the Tools: Circles, Maps and Paths.* Toronto: Inclusion Press; L. Jordan and C. Goodey (1996). *Human Rights and School Change.* Bristol: CSIE.

2   Exclusion

Jonny, Micah and Tej can look at each other and each knows what the other one is going to do next. They delight in joke routines. They high-five, do man hugs and ask each other what they've been doing. They call round uninvited bringing beers and invite each other to birthday parties. They are in their twenties and all in paid employment – one in the motor trade, one on a city farm and one in theatre design. They would all be upset if one of them lost touch; they give to each other, and appreciate what the other gives. Jonny, the common friend (Micah and Tej see each other less often), is particularly funny and charismatic. Those close to him say 'it's an honour to receive his attention'. He is delighted in turn when he sees the others. He speaks less by using words than by making trilling noises and dancing up and down on the spot or rushing round the room. Micah and Tej have known him since they were at school together. Micah met him in primary school. When he was ten, he brought his new bike round to show Jonny – so when he passed his driving test Jonny was the first person he drove round to, to show him the car. Jonny met Tej at secondary school, a highly successful flagship comprehensive in East London. Jonny's mother facilitated visits when they were younger. Now they choose to be with each other. They are natural and unembarrassed when doing ordinary or extraordinary things outside the house.

That is what friendship is, as distinct from doing boy scout duties or volunteering. At the start of this century, the UK became the first country in the world to promote friendship as a policy goal – in fact its chief policy goal alongside deinstitutionalization and ordinary lives, and the more familiar 'rights' and 'independence' – for adults with learning difficulties.[1] This was greeted with scepticism and some resistance from institutions on the ground, from professionals and administrators across to voluntary organizations and even the advocacy movement. Negative criticism in the academy has likewise come from across the range, from radicals to conservatives. I do not see it as my job to defend principles that assume the full humanity of everyone, and I shall not be doing so here. Nor, however, having nodded approval of the policy, am I going to pass hastily on to anticipate its failure in practice. The eventual outcomes of policy will depend on the nuts and bolts of future local activity, which lie outside the scope of this book. It is not simply the case that governments issue a policy and people carry it out. Individual aspects of it may break off and have an influence on their own, or get turned inside out and *then* have an influence, or get lost completely. Instead, my main object for analysis is that resistance mentality, together with its long historical context and possible future ones.

Being sceptical about received opinion is a necessary starting-point for research of any kind. But being sceptical about *policy* can sometimes be a screen for *lack* of scepticism about the basic concepts one is using, which is a more difficult business. For example, there are those who regard the policy as a 'recipe for failure' because it 'excludes' the more profoundly disabled. In what way does it exclude them? Because, it is said, they are not capable of friendship.[2] Admittedly, the authors go on to qualify this with the phrase 'friendship as commonly understood'. But who is it that forms this commonalty? Centuries ago, the peer community of normal, cognitive capacity was defined by possession of what were known as 'the common ideas' – a set of unchanging principles covering philosophy, mathematics and religion. It was the community that considered itself the intellectual elite inasmuch as it was also the gently born social elite. The cognitively deficient, those who did not possess the common ideas, were thus a good 75 per cent of the population. Today's population, now explained not so much by their lack of ideas as their lack of the psychological mechanisms behind them, are a tiny 1 per cent or so. But in both cases their definition as deficient comes down to ingroup members' mutual recognition of each other as a distinct community.

The historical example is important because it enables us to see present criticism of the policy as circular. We shall come across many circularities in the course of this book. What is friendship 'as commonly understood'? That which a profoundly learning disabled person cannot understand. What is a profoundly learning disabled person? Someone who cannot understand friendship as commonly understood. Seen in this light, the accusation that this particular government policy excludes people seems to be a projection of the critics' own urge to exclude, just as the medieval elite did.

Take another policy goal, paid employment. James came out of a long-stay institution with 'complex needs', an IQ below 40 and a reputation for aggression and waywardness. The normal route would have been for him to go into sheltered housing and day services. His paid supporters warned that paid employment was not suitable for someone like James, who carried such a long list of negatives. In any case, they had not asked him if he wanted it; as is so often the case, the anger that fuelled his aggression was precisely the result of his not being listened to or valued. And it turned out that he wanted to work. He now has two part-time jobs amounting to full time, at a legal wage. One fulfils his manual skills, which he uses to help look after the appearance of a large and precious Tudor building. The other is as a greeter at the forecourt and cafe of a large recreational site where young children and families visit. He is adept at making them feel comfortable and at home, and his particular sense of humour is just right. The necessary 'reasonable adjustments' required for both jobs under equalities legislation turn out to be minimal; on occasions when he leaves his post because he is feeling bad, he is told to get back on the job because he is getting paid for it, and he does so.

Those with conservative values, especially in the medical arena, who consider learning disability a disease, assume it to be a self-evident absurdity that someone like James could hold down a properly paid job. Actually, though, he does. And if he can, why can't anyone else like him? Meanwhile, for many radical social theorists opposed to that medical model, the goal of paid employment is anathema because it is an example of capitalism gone mad. They assume that people like James are being *forced* to *compete* for jobs. It seems as if they are offering a critique of neo-liberal economics, but as we shall see later it is James who in this instance is offering the more fundamental critique.

Surely a policy that can unite the strangest of bedfellows in opposition must be wrong? Either that, or something else is going on. Ordinary lives demand ordinary people. Are those labelled with learning disabilities really not ordinary people? Not like the rest of us? And what would lead you or me to hold that position? The idea that everyone means everyone does not amount to holding a position at all. It goes without saying. It does not require justification. People are people. A position is only taken – the first move is made – by someone who feels like drawing boundaries. The onus is on that person, the one who thinks there needs to be some sort of subclassification within the realm of what we habitually call human. What accounts for that urge? A cynical answer might be that the disparate objectors are united by their reliance on a concept of learning disability which they assume to be stable and without which they would either be out of work or forced to change their ways. But self-interest cannot be the final explanation. Salary, professional status or simply being too lazy to think through what one is doing are never more than pointers to something deeper. Moreover we can also count within the professions (and perhaps even the academy) on some fearless individuals trying to remedy injustice and break down barriers of segregation and exclusion.

Outgroups and their boundaries

What is ordinary life? Of course it is different in different eras and places, and we shall be looking here at our own. The possibility that in talking about people with learning difficulties we might be talking about ordinary people, and the stimulus for recognizing this in UK policy and legislation, has come from the people who know them best: from families, and in more recent history from advocates and professionals concerned with the closure of long-stay hospitals.

Why then are some ordinary people not wanted? The next two chapters will show how unstable and transitory a concept learning disability is, but it still needs a working definition. And defining a concept demands that we look at it first in context, alongside other comparable concepts, before trying to say what it is in and of itself. My initial approach to the question above, then, is to consider what other disorders of mind and behaviour are related to learning disability, and how. The very fact that we have such a concept is evidence for a general disorder that seems to run across societies and results in the creation of social outgroups. Let's call it inclusion phobia, if only because inclusion is a familiar term that features in current policy-making. True, inclusion is now referred to in so many social and political contexts as to seem nebulous and suspect. But in the learning disability field it has quite separate origins that are very specific. Here inclusion was coined to describe the optimum outcome of the closure of segregated institutions. To regard it as suspect in this field too, by transference – to hint that no such thing can be or actually is being practised in formal social institutions such as employment, education or other aspects of people's social lives – is a prevarication, itself typical of inclusion phobia. As for that word phobia, it may be objected that my use of it here is just satirical, or at best a rhetorical flourish aimed at making the thing sound more scientific than it really is. Even if that were the case, it would be no more rhetorical or less scientific than most other existing psychiatric categories.

One could easily argue that an urge to exclude is displayed towards outgroups of all sorts, not only people with learning difficulties. These various specific urges have something in common: they are all projections of anxiety not only on to the *object* of fear, to the physical presence of outgroup members, but also to their *objectification*, that is, to the initial process of conceptualizing them as a group. Not just broad theories of marginalization but the entire record of anthropological research shows that such ingroup/outgroup patterns, along with their exclusionary mentalities, are a structural feature of all complex societies. Especially with the passage of time, the patterns can seem arbitrary. Take racism. If it persists today it is because, as experiments in social psychology have suggested, differences in skin colour, though inessential in themselves, are so obvious to the naked eye that they just happen to be a convenient trigger for reinforcing a prior, colour-blind desire to maintain existing ingroup/outgroup structures of some more material kind (networks of wealth, professional status, etc.).[3] That is to say: differences based on skin colour are not essential to the social structures of Western societies today, but nor are they the mere residue of the bygone structures to which they *were* once essential.

By contrast, learning disability *does* have an essential relationship to present structures. It provokes a pathological state which ingroups arrive at only sometimes: a war footing, where the objective is to annihilate the threat which a particular group represents to the ingroup's own core idea of who they are. The target in such cases is not just any outgroup but a special case: what I shall call, to borrow a term, an *extreme* outgroup.[4] Hence the attempt to eliminate outgroup members or potential members, as an underlying principle. Physical impairment may be similar in this respect (AFP tests for spina bifida are a case in point); but supposed bodily perfection is less intrinsic to modern ideal forms of self-representation because unlike learning disability it does not place a question mark over a person's species membership. Nor am I indulging in special pleading for people with learning difficulties as against others marginalized on similarly 'intellectual' grounds such as old people with dementia or the long-term mentally ill, to whom much of what I am saying is also relevant. It is the birth-to-death identity of learning disability that lies at the heart of inclusion phobia; it is the vortex that sucks down those other groups with them, and is therefore the one that needs to be dealt with.

Inclusion phobia in action

Extreme pathological fear may seem an exaggerated description of everyday events. When the young man behind the bank counter pleasantly asks me, about the person I am with, 'Can he sign his name?' is it really equivalent to our fear of the alien that just jumped out of John Hurt's chest? Yes. Both constitute a recognition that there are 'perilous substances ... dreadful bits of otherness which manage somehow to insinuate themselves at the core of one's being'.[5] The phobia can be mild, but it is still a phobia.

In terms of social organization it has more severe effects than that. Inclusion phobia in action displays many of the features of narcissistic bullying directed at any seemingly weaker individual naïve enough to seek parity, a lightning skill for mendacity, and an ability to represent these as rational. Take the village primary school that meets with the parents of six-year-old Alisha. The headteacher says it does not have the extra human resources to 'meet Alisha's needs'. The parents report visiting a school in another area, which said it would be happy to have Alisha within its existing arrangements. Should they be forced to move house? Ignoring this response, the headteacher then says her presence will be detrimental to the other children. For example, 'She won't be able to sit still in assembly'. Her parents ask how many six-year-olds do. Without pause or answer the headteacher moves sideways again. The school will need building works, a changing room; the embarrassed local authority adviser calls her bluff and suggests the authority might provide it. The headteacher therefore jumps to a speech about there being two segregated (special) schools in the area that would be so much better for Alisha, and offers to set up visits for the parents. The parents are driven to ask, 'Why don't you want her here?' to which the headteacher says repeatedly, 'Oh but we *do* want her here. Why do you keep saying that?' The parents decline her offer, though the unsolicited appointments arrive anyway.

The parents' first reaction is that the school is being unreasonable. But even this is an inadequate description, itself rooted in the same dominant ideology that excludes her. The school's reaction to Alisha is not unreasonable, it is insane. Observe the behaviour more closely. Typically objection *a*, once satisfactorily met, will jump to objection *b* and likewise to *c* and so on (often returning to *a* again, as if it had not already been dealt with), without any connection between them other than their source in the phobia itself. The answer to the question about the school not wanting her is clearly schizoid. The word unreasonable suggests, not lack of sanity, but that the offending party can be reasoned out of such a pattern of bullying by referring them to some universally accepted norm. In cases like Alisha's, however, that will not work, because reason itself, and universally accepted norms in general, exist by virtue of the *a priori* exclusion of people like her. The headteacher's behaviour meets psychiatry's formal definitional criteria for anxiety disorder and specific phobia: namely, that 'the anxiety must be out of proportion to the actual danger or threat ... *after cultural contextual factors are taken into account*' [my italics].[6]

In the case of inclusion phobia, that 'cultural context' is the entire modern era and its dominant ideology. That is why equalities law in this field, whatever the letter of it, rarely achieves what persuasion has failed to achieve. Parents or advocates pursuing inclusion will recognize the frustration here, at an institution's evidently non-negotiable position. And contrary to the platitude that inclusion is only for children of university educated professionals like Alisha's who can negotiate the system, it is in fact harder for them; they are more likely to have imbibed those rational norms, so resisting the irrationality of segregation is harder and more shocking than it is for working-class people. Most parents, of whatever social class, having received the phobia's negative messages from day one of diagnosis, either do not even realize that legally their child is entitled to a place in the local school whatever her difficulties, or abandon the idea at the slightest hint of equivocation from it. However, working-class parents, if they get as far as Alisha's, are at least more likely to recognize street-level bullying when they see it. In practice, the best way for an ally or advocate to stiffen the sinews has always been to remind the parents of what is already deeply felt knowledge: *you're* not mad, *they* are. The very act of demanding a place where all the other local children are, grounded as it is in the reality of the child's full species membership, constitutes a challenge to the sufferer's delusion to the contrary – a challenge that unfortunately tends to provoke further negative stereotyping of the excluded individual.

Historical change and 'radical evil'

Before the modern era the extreme outgroups were different, as we shall see; more than one could be conceived or targeted at the same time; and they tended to be localized. Today the power of the phobia is reinforced by the global reach and significance of its core concern, which is the human intellect. The very idea of a universal human nature defined by a species-specific intellect was the novel founding principle of the modern era, from the eighteenth-century Enlightenment onwards. Yet from the beginning, this view of what it is to be human bore within itself, necessarily, its own particular way of fashioning and rejecting others. The idea of learning disability and of a person thus disabled is the distilled essence of this. The Enlightenment's friendliest critic, Immanuel Kant, could already see that the idealization of human reason might be an excuse for abusing others; he clearly thought this latter tendency might be some permanent condition of humanity (he called it 'radical evil', seeing it as the secular equivalent of original sin).[7]

The concept of learning disability, as the modern era's own expression of inclusion phobia, is nevertheless the culmination of a process whose roots lie further back than the Enlightenment. Its characteristics have derived from those of other outgroups that have come and gone in tandem with changes in the ingroup and its self-appointed characteristics, while inclusion phobia has remained the continuing factor. That is why the latter has to be the starting-point for knowing anything about its more temporary phenomena, of which learning disability is just one. In the search for stable knowledge in our field, it provides the most long-lasting historical foundation we can find. By comparison with inclusion phobia, learning disability itself, being a recent and unstable category, is an unreliable conceptual tool for present-day practice.

This is not disability denial. As materialist histories of physical disability demonstrate too, it is not mere concepts but actual complexities of economic and social organization that create the kind of person who is disabled from negotiating them and who may need support in order to belong.[8] In this respect, people were right to criticize the anti-psychiatry movement of the 1960s and 1970s for putting mental illness under a purely social category such as 'deviancy', or worse, an 'alternative lifestyle'. What mentally ill people have to fear is not 'wanton intervention' but neglect.[9] However, learning disability is something else again. In this case wanton intervention, in the form of separate (special) provision and exclusion from the ordinary life of mainstream social institutions, *is* neglect. Certainly all the long-term historical transformations in the casting and re-casting of extreme outgroups make it reasonable to ask: what is real about learning disability? Even if it cannot be dismissed as just an alternative lifestyle, were any such people recognized in the distant past?

The answer, as I have suggested, is No. Even if that were not the case, the fact that the question remains largely unasked is itself indicative. What we do know is that classifying a human group by intellectual criteria is today's prevailing symptom of inclusion phobia. Intellectual disability is vital to the dominant ingroup because of its relationship to the quality which that group, as currently constituted, attributes to itself *and which it therefore employs as its core definition of the human species as a whole.* Intellectual ability, or intelligence, is in modern societies the foremost claim to status based on permanent inner attributes, as distinct from temporary outward ones such as power or wealth. As a subjective possession, personal intelligence is seen to correspond with the neutral, objective and permanent rationality of these societies' scientific knowledge systems. There has always been something convenient, not to say magical, about the way the sciences of the mind get these two realms, subjective and objective, to match up. Intelligence, like other ingroup qualities of the past, entails an extreme group in which that quality is incurably absent, and the absence scientifically demonstrable. Yet historical research shows that the intelligence is a historically contingent notion. It is not a natural human property that has simply been represented in different ways across history. It is of itself a new arrival: a form of cultural self-representation that grew from and usurped earlier forms of self-representation. The same therefore must go for intellectual disability, the negative status marker.

In its motivations inclusion phobia is narcissistic. In lieu of genuine objectivity the definition of a property such as intelligence and likewise the definition of its absence can only be modelled on the self-determined characteristics and standpoint of the person doing the defining. The mundane behaviours exhibited by the phobia – gossip, discrimination, scapegoating, accusatory bullying, segregation, and physical elimination or prevention – are strong and taken for granted in modern social structures. They occur in situations of inequality generally, but with the extreme outgroup they display their especially pathological nature by being in inverse proportion to the size and capacity of the population targeted. The mere request by someone to be included in what everyone else does often induces a mad anger, which will be recognizable to anyone who has been in Alisha's position. Her parents' willingness to persist means they are only a small group within an already small minority ('profoundly' disabled) within the small learning disabled minority – but that group's experience is normal.

Beware of ethics

To repeat: this book does not adopt an ethical standpoint and is not about ethics at all. It is no good wishing narcissistic bullies would be nicer to you. Before that can happen, there is a need to analyse, understand and predict their behaviour. Ethical debates, as presently constituted, only hinder that analysis. My focus will be on sanity. Bioethics and philosophical ethics in general, inasmuch as they are perceived to be specially relevant to the field, are themselves partly the product of inclusion phobia. They are only present because a tacit question has already been raised. To be or not to be? It can only be answered with another and prior question: why should such an existential issue arise in the first place? Ethics, as a discipline, does not hang around in the air for most lives or potential lives. The answer is: only because of the existence already of an underlying urge to exclude, irrespective of the object of exclusion, which is a moveable feast.

Modern debates about life and death, in relation to people with learning difficulties and where physical suffering does not apply, emerge *from within* the phobia; they are intrinsic to an irrational complex in which ethical justifications, biological knowledge and psychological presuppositions are folded into each other. The same is true at the other end of the intelligence spectrum, where an ethical stance is already encoded in the very nature of genetic enhancement, superintelligence and transhumanism.[10] The roots of this complex lie, as we shall see later, in medieval theology and its theories of the immortality of the soul. For the moment let us ask: who are the conservatives here? The impression given is that those who resist genetic enhancement and elimination are. In fact quite the opposite may be true.

The specifically modern and 'extreme' element in bioethics appears in the way we separate ethics from morals and even set them in opposition to each other. In fact they are the same word, the first Greek the second Latin, for what was once one and the same debate: namely, what is the good life. The Greeks' answer, by contrast with today's greatest happiness principle, was roughly that it is 'the way we do things here' (that is why they also provide the etymological root for our words 'ethos' and 'mores'). In the remote academic heights this remains the case. The exam paper one university philosophy department calls ethics another calls moral philosophy and vice-versa. In common usage, however, ethics has now become the term used to describe how medicine, official public discourse, and the law frame a decision, while morals tends to be the term applied to decisions that buck the trend: lay, private, unreasonable. The medical profession in particular, aided by media prominence given the Pro-Life movement, tends to spin this by referring it to the debate between science and faith, imputing religious motives to 'moral' decisions. The elevation of ethics into a system of political brokerage of human existence and non-existence is the marginalization of morals. Ethics belongs to power, morals to a regrettable heterodoxy.

A paired example will suffice. It is September 2012. The abortion debate, as tepid in the UK as it is hot in the USA, stirs briefly: the British Secretary of State for Health has aired the idea of restricting the legal time-limit to within 12 weeks, on the grounds that only 9 per cent of abortions occur later and are usually due to the discovery of Down's syndrome. In fact the law already allows an exception in such cases, which therefore means, for him, 'In that case, it's OK' – exactly as it does for the right-to-choose movement whose anger he has sparked. In that same week *The Archers*, a notoriously middle-of-the road radio soap, features 46-year-old Vicky who, pregnant with her first child, learns that it has Down's syndrome and wants to give birth. The baby's arrival ushers in a positive storyline (religion is not mentioned). In the respective media discussions that follow, the secretary of state's decision is about ethics, Vicky's about her morals.

Ethical debates as currently framed are a diversion from the prior task, which is to find a firm knowledge base. So where do we look for one? If learning disability is a medium-term historical contingency and the more essential, long-lasting pathology is that tendency of a phobic dominant ideology to create extreme albeit unstable outgroups as a way of valorizing itself, is there an existing theory that would help us understand how it works?

Inclusion phobia, contamination disgust and fear of pollution

Possible elements for a coherent theory of inclusion phobia are scattered across various fields. The various approaches, which we are going to look at in more detail, can contribute to a stable knowledge base because they all hint at the historical permanence of the disorder, and because all of them locate what is wrong not in the extreme outgroup but in the ingroup. Some but not all the authors go so far as to suggest, like Kant, that the disorder is rooted in human nature. Typically, inclusion phobia exhibits an urge both to categorize other people and to create real-life institutions and practices; the conceptual and social segregation are mutually interdependent processes. None of the authors, though, mentions learning disability as a case in point, let alone *the* case – a limitation certainly, and perhaps itself a symptom.

DSM5 lists fear of contamination and dirt under obsessive compulsive disorder. Stanley Rachman, the leading authority on OCD, describes it as 'extraordinarily persistent, variable ... culturally accepted and even prescribed', and as we shall see constantly with regard to both learning disability and intelligence, 'tinged with magical thinking'. It can 'be established without [having any actual] physical contact' with dirty, impure things or with 'people regarded as untouchables (culturally or personally defined)'. Those affected by the phobia may 'seal off parts of their homes and even lock up rooms that contain contaminated material'.[11] The symptoms, then, are inseparably individual and social. Obsessive individuals seal off their homes, obsessive societies seal off their ordinary institutions – the places where we study, work and interact socially.

Disgust, which is closely associated with fear of contamination, seems to be chiefly a group disorder.[12] Anthropologists such as Mary Douglas have identified this fear of dirt as the organizing principle in recognizing anomaly, across all societies.[13] It leads to 'anxiety and from there to suppression or avoidance', and hence to socio-cultural 'rituals of separation'. Douglas's maxim runs: fear of dirt is universal but what is considered dirt changes. Her widely known work has been applied to many topics. As she herself says, the notion of dirt is 'a kind of omnibus compendium which includes all the rejected elements of ordered systems'. All you have to do, it seems, is identify something people like to steer clear of and then put it down to their fear of dirt. At the applied level, then, her theory is a key that will open any door, not specific enough to account on its own for learning disability. In fact she does not mention it. Ironically, it is precisely the failure of any of the approaches discussed here to identify it as one of their examples of extreme otherness that corroborates another of Douglas's important principles, namely, that fear of impurity is an *unconscious* common denominator of social practices and group mentalities. Clearly, then, that goes for the mentality of the human sciences themselves. Certain functions link all extreme outgroups, particularly that of reinforcing the ingroup's self-esteem and codifying its own status; so, through a concept such as intellectual disability, the ingroup justifies and rationalizes its own disorder to itself. However, in attempting to define this disability specifically, we need to distinguish its characteristics more clearly from the generality of other excluded groups.

Feelings of disgust towards people with learning difficulties derive from feelings of disgust about animals and animality. These feelings are not necessarily a universal human characteristic, as they seem not to be universally present in non-Western cultures. Fear of animals is one of DSM's main subdivisions of specific phobia, and is linked to fear of death. Research in which people are prompted with reminders of death has shown that their fears can be correlated with an increased reaction of disgust at animals. The need of human beings to distinguish themselves from other animals springs from an anxiety about their own mortality; animality reminds them about this and is therefore threatening.[14] Disgust, especially at members of the same species, seems not to occur in other animals.[15] Under experimental conditions, extreme outgroup clusters are perceived to be less than human, or fully non-human. One of the clusters in this study was disabled people. (The experiment did not distinguish between physical and intellectual disability and was based on subjects' viewing of visual images which naturally exhibit physical features better than cognitive ones.[16]) We shall see later how such feelings have previous origins in the medieval idea of the ladder of nature. The abstract desire of modern societies for the human race to develop towards increasing intellectual perfection can be seen as an expression and continuation of this.

Rachman recognizes 'associations between the [individual] fear of contamination and social fears and phobias'. Social psychologists such as Henri Tajfel go further, insisting that individual states of mind are not 'bricks from which an adequate social psychology can be built: the derivations [of outgroup theory are] in the opposite direction'.[17] Douglas's theory of purity and danger takes us further still. It helps us to see the conceptualization of learning disability as one piece of evidence for a collective disorder (one might say psychosis) which expresses itself in obsessive attempts to verify its fear that out there, in the darkness always just beyond the searchlight of pathology, is a gathering invasion of dirt, embodied in an army of creatures who are only pretending to be human and who must therefore be precisely tracked, categorized, subcategorized, labelled, assessed, segregated, and eliminated. And what Douglas regards as a structural feature can also be traced as a historical process. The actual traits of this group – the crucial features that have filled the extreme outgroup template over time – slowly but surely change and in the long term are transformed utterly.

Inclusion phobia as false consciousness

Some psychiatrists, identifying 'false consciousness' as a core symptom of schizophrenia, have seen it not only as an individual disorder but also as a group one, typical of powerful ingroups. Joseph Gabel studied under Eugène Minkowski, an early authority on schizophrenia and former assistant of Eugen Bleuler (inventor of the terms schizophrenia and autism). He describes how alongside the characteristic paranoid delusions and split thinking of the schizoid disorders, false consciousness displays human thought paralysed and frozen in time, in an 'autistic' state abstracted from reality. Linking the personal to the political, Gabel diagnoses a 'schizophrenic structure of ideological thought' in the dominant ideologies of modern capitalist society.[18] The denial of history is necessary to these regimes, since any awareness of major historical change would expose the 'fatuity' of their privileged, ingroup world view and reveal that they were merely temporary occupants of its restricted social niche. It is not just that ruling elites manipulate history to suit their own agendas. All economically and politically dominant ingroups suffer from the same kind of dysfunction as the individual schizophrenic, exhibiting 'thought enclosed within itself ... unchanged by experience'. The ingroup's view of what is socially normal, then, corresponds with the relentless 'logic of schizophrenia' in the individual psyche. Another way of putting this is to say that each individual member of the dominant ingroup is 'caught up in the "logic" of ... persecution from the persecutor's standpoint, and cannot break away'.[19] This logic, says Gabel, ignores the experience of 'lived time'. In shutting down the temporal dimensions of thought, it blanks out the prospect of radical future change.

This disordered, excess logic involves a lopsided emphasis on classification and labelling. If we think about this in terms of an intelligent ingroup (that is, the group of all those with normal intelligence and above), we can begin to see how inclusion phobia can take the form of delusions exhibiting themselves through the psychology of intelligence. The more evidence-based they are, the more delusional they are: a symptom of 'morbid rationalism' and of what Gabel, following Minkowski, calls an excess of 'the identificatory function'. It dresses these up as 'the normal,' allowing the latter to take on a 'social sacredness' that 'lives under the sign of identity', where identity is fixed and non-temporal.[20] It is true that labelling can sometimes 'start off as a healthy limiting concept', but it ends up as a 'universe eternally immutable'. Here again the characteristics of this social disorder correspond with the 'delusional, autistic' state of the schizophrenic's individual disorder.

Although Gabel's Marxist view of history as dialectic tells him the ultimate outgroup is the proletariat, the one he most often cites here is the one that inspired his researches, the Jews in Nazi Europe. Racist false consciousness denies history by building a 'pseudo-history' which, instead of explaining the Jews through their historical arrival and the gradual construction of a Jewish identity, 'claims to explain history through the Jew'. We could say, similarly, that explanatory claims about human nature (as human intelligence) can only be made through positing a fixed intellectually disabled identity that exists in nature and needs to be fought against. Such a claim is implicit in evolutionary psychology, cognitive genetics and bioethics, and across the range of the human sciences in general.

Nevertheless, there are limits to how far false consciousness theory can help us understand inclusion phobia. Gabel cannot escape the restricted perspective of modernism, which distorts historical time by enshrining it in individual development and social progress. A perspective like this is clearly incapable of interrogating present concepts of intellectual disability, which is defined precisely by the fact that it *hinders* development and progress. Gabel's Marxism was of the humanist variety that emphasizes history and time over structural permanence, but it takes away with one hand what it delivers with the other. It asserts that human nature, albeit universal, is not immutable and cross-historical, but reproduces and changes, as particular outcomes of particular eras.[21] This apparently Marxist formula, which actually goes back to the Enlightenment, assumes that the overall effect of change is progressive, tending towards social and therefore intellectual perfection as the next stage in history. A negative like disability clearly does not belong in this picture.

Moreover, Gabel's only historical example of false consciousness turns out to be contemporary with himself. The paradigmatic outgroup targeted by false consciousness is a racial and religious other. However, the centrality of intelligence and thus intellectual disability in modern societies is such that the Holocaust, with its roots in late medieval anti-semitism (when the Jews were indeed an extreme outgroup), can be seen rather as a temporary digression from that broader historical trend, within which Nazism was a deviant and only spuriously 'rational' anomaly. Gabel is more interested in history as dialectic – a broad theoretical axiom – than in specifying concrete changes in a shifting multiplicity of ingroup/outgroup relations. What his account of false consciousness does none the less provide, even though it does not mention intelligence or learning disability, is some analytical tools for understanding how disability arrived among us and has come to be defined the way it is.

Inclusion phobia and the great incarceration

Another perspective on inclusion phobia could come from the already well established genre of the history of segregated institutions, though in fact it gives us a somewhat restricted and distorting picture. Even at their modern height, let alone in the middle ages, these institutions did not incarcerate the majority of adults labelled with learning disability or anything like it. The basic entry criterion for a medieval almshouse or lazar house was poverty more than intelligence.[22] In any case these were partly mainstream institutions, since they were open to and involved in the society's commercial and social networks.[23] It is modern historians who have promoted the theme of sheer physical separateness, mirroring our own segregationist values. And most importantly, the launching-point for modern historical theory has been an entirely different category, the mentally ill. The psychiatrist Jacques Lacan claimed that the madman who thinks he is a king is no crazier than the king who thinks he is a king, but even in such radical circles it would be thought highly unusual, or mere playfulness, to add: the person with learning difficulties who thinks he is intelligent is no stupider than the intelligent person who thinks he is intelligent. Even though the history of mental illness has led by association to a sub-genre of the institutional history of people with learning difficulties, it ignores the quite separate and distinctive nature of their *conceptual* history. An exception can be made of some historians who have pointed out how important it is that many nineteenth- and twentieth-century inmates were there partly on grounds of their social class or personal economic circumstances.[24] But it still leaves open the idea that the category of learning disability itself indicates a cross-historical natural kind.

The Foucauldian theory of a 'great incarceration' as a grand historical moment may be lopsided, but it has a role in accounting for inclusion phobia because it too argues that 'the explanation [has] to be sought not among the victims, but among the persecutors', and that this forces us to confront the political face of the phobia.[25] Shoring up Foucault's rather ramshackle approach to history with some actual scholarship, R. I. Moore has revealed the medieval antecedents of institutional segregation as the start of 'the formation of a persecutory society'. On the one hand, the codification of extreme outgroups – in this case Jews, heretics and lepers – was becoming tighter, while on the other hand the conceptual characteristics describing such groups remained loose enough to meander from one group to another. Moore sees the persecuting ingroup as a unified power, a type that exists prior to any construction of particular types of outgroup. Its impulse is to create receptacles for its phobias about 'filth, stench and putrefaction', and the Devil. Consequently ghettoization, sequestration of property, disinheritance, and ultimately physical liquidation – the brute facts of social administration – are the shared fate of all such groups, imposed by an ingroup in whose own mental disorder the final explanation must be sought.[26]

Moore takes the important step of aiming at a precise periodization. If the urge to persecute and the consequent firming up of categories became more intense after 1200 AD, this was not just a gradual evolution out of some vague Dark Ages barbarism but a concrete juncture in the economic and cultural history of Western Europe. I argue in the next chapter that the beginnings of this trend lie somewhat further back, with the growth of Empire among the later Romans. Nevertheless, whatever the precise dating, to organize detail it is necessary to establish major landmarks, and the late middle ages was one of them.

Moore identifies the new set of ingroup characteristics in this period as those of a rising literate clerical caste. The *literati* (effectively this meant literate in Latin) were the first generation to have been educated in the first universities. Their theological and philosophical studies defined what goes on in the human mind as a process of logical reasoning, information-processing and the making of abstractions – a list of items which, though familiar enough to a modern cognitive scientist, was then novel. But not coincidental. Those were precisely the skills that many of them would apply in their subsequent day jobs, as clerks meeting the rapidly expanding bureaucratic requirements of church and state administration. Abstraction and information-processing, after all, are a kind of mental filing (as illustrated today by all those odd-one-out questions in intelligence tests). Was there not a place among medieval outgroups, then, for a human category defined by the *in*ability to reason logically, to abstract or to process information? One that would therefore correspond to modern, cognitive definitions of disability? It would surely have been an obvious projection of their own skills, for the clerical caste to make.

The medieval term *idiota* was not equivalent to our own; all it signified was someone who could not write or perhaps read, or even any lay person.[27] In the courts it applied in a more technical sense to a certain type of incompetence, though obviously that would only entail people of sufficient standing to have affairs that demanded competence as a matter of record; it was therefore not a cognitive definition as such. Moreover, as Moore (perhaps unwittingly) indicates, it was not sharply distinguished from mental illness. Medieval law did not define a category that corresponds precisely with today's learning disability, and although signs of some conceptual shift towards it can sometimes be detected, retrospective diagnosis is tricky business.[28] Several centuries were needed before a separate and pure solution of idiocy would be precipitated from the medieval concoction of loosely bounded human labels whose characteristics were often interchangeable from one to another. The clerical caste might secondarily ascribe deficiencies in logical reasoning and abstraction to Jews, heretics and lepers, and even more to the laity in general, but these common characteristics did not yet define a cognitive type on its own. Nevertheless, clerical stereotypes were the start of something significant.

Moore's sociological and institutional approach, like the other theories cited in this chapter, takes us some way towards an explanation for inclusion phobia, but without a forward reference to learning disability it is incomplete. It would be in keeping with social theory's focus on marginalized people to say that only those with learning difficulties themselves can go the whole way to explaining inclusion phobia. However, they are absent not only from mainstream institutions, and not only from the academic community, but from social theory itself. What might Foucault's view of them have been? Even Moore is struck by 'his readiness to accept for the leper houses of medieval Europe the positivist account of their history and functions that he had rejected for the lunatic asylums which took their place'.[29] If Foucault had ever been asked how he saw learning disability, it would either have to be in a positive medical slot (a disease, as the medical profession still largely conceives it) along with leprosy, or as an undifferentiated sub-set of mental illness. Social theory has thus not dealt with the *specificity* of learning disability.

While the historical perspective of a great incarceration over the last two centuries has been also a great awakening, its ahistorical weakness is that it reduces specific outgroup categories to a mélange of marginalizations in which the core distinctiveness of learning disability and the fate of people categorized in this way, and therefore the best shot at identifying and explaining modern inclusion phobia across the board, are lost.

Inclusion phobia and the scapegoat mechanism

Another feature of inclusion phobia is what anthropologists call the scapegoat mechanism. This concept has been employed to explain how the persecution of outgroups is an attempt to deny mortality and how linguistic symbols create negative stereotypes as a way of raising the status of the stereotyper;[30] in René Girard's work, which has a religious strand, it describes how scapegoating offers the prospect of cure, on the grounds that it is only inclusion of the once-scapegoated victim that can effect social healing.[31] The scapegoat is not just another Other. Girard's theory aims at specificity, at a 'typology of the stereotypes of persecution'.[32] It is also a teleological theory: that is, its future is contained and predicted in its present. This time we are heading somewhere: not Power is Everywhere, more the Book of Revelation. The scapegoat myths which Girard reviews, from the Old Testament's Job via Sophocles's Oedipus to Wagner's Parsifal, show that religion is important to explaining inclusion phobia because it holds out the prospect of salvation.

The themes of contamination by dirt, poison, bestiality or monstrosity ('confusion of animals and men') occur frequently in mythology. The theory of a scapegoat mechanism is useful inasmuch as it focuses clearly on the most extreme outgroups. Girard explains their formation as resulting from a 'crisis of differentiation'. Persecutors are convinced that a tiny number of people, despite their weakness, can ruin a whole society.[33] The scapegoat mechanism is a projection of the animosity between the rival groups of a society on to a smaller group that is consequently expelled and persecuted. This is necessary at crisis points when the contending parties in a community become 'undif-ferentiated, deprived of all that distinguishes one person from another in time and space', with the result that 'all are equally disordered in the same place and at the same time'. Douglas too says that 'pollution dangers strike when form has been attacked'.[34]

Whereas the Foucauldians tend to see the late middle ages as the arrival of something nastier (a stricter urge to classify) out of a previously loose system of categorizations, scapegoating theory sees green shoots of renewal. In the early modern era, it says, belief in occult forces starts to wane; the search for someone to blame continues, but 'looks for a more substantial cause ... The lightweight quality of magic as a cause is anchored to materiality and there-fore to "scientific" logic'.[35] One example is alchemy, whose magical, 'demoniac' elements early scientists succeeding in tying to the material world, and which became what we now know as chemistry. It is certainly confirmed in the learning disability field by pre-natal diagnosis, where a historical residue of devil beliefs is anchored, not dissipated, by present-day genetic explanations.[36] At the same time, says Girard, we are now all on the way to being cured of our scapegoating urges. With his interest in mass salvation, Girard is the only one of these theorists to look into the crystal ball. 'A formidable revolution is about to take place', he says.[37] Over the course of European history 'repre-sentations of persecution from the persecutor's standpoint gradually weaken and disappear'. Moreover, his shining example is our increased social acceptance of the disabled. He does not distinguish between physical and learning dis-ability here. It seems the latter has not occurred to him; for example, although *Parsifal* is about a scapegoat who turns into a saviour, Girard omits to say that Parsifal starts life as a nameless fool.

Like the other theories, Girard's is hampered by this lacuna. He writes about the persecutor's perspective being 'imposed' over others. However, learning disability is hardly a perspective at all, imposed or otherwise, it is, as it seems to us, a quasi-universal truth. The persecutor is the intelligence society as a whole, that is, the 99 per cent of the population not learning disabled. Girard sees an equivalence between the inherently religious promise of his theory, as cure or salvation, and the rise of modern science's search for natural causes:

'To lead men to the patient exploration of natural causes, men must first be turned away from their victims, and this can only be done by showing them that from now on persecutors "hate without cause"'. Yet 'hating without cause' seems a perfectly adequate description of what modern science's biotechnicians and segregating social administrators routinely do in relation to learning disability. The category of people incapable of scientific inquiry into natural causes, because of their lack of the logical, abstracting and information-processing abilities that constitute such inquiry, is the ghost in the scapegoat mechanism.

Inclusion phobia and experimental verification

With Girard's quasi-religious anthropological theory we seem to have drifted a long way from the phobia's scientific profile, with which we started out. So let us see if we can tie it back down. Rachman and DSM5 describe a version of inclusion phobia in individuals. Can *experimental* psychology do this for *groups*?

In even the most basic of mental operations – in the act of perception, for example – values are a contributory, organizing factor, as a seminal paper, moreover one dealing largely with intelligence, demonstrated half a century ago.[38] On this basis experimental researchers subsequently succeeding in finding that the more extreme the instance of an observed outgroup category, the more accessible it is to memory retrieval. Since it is more striking and therefore over-represented in an ingroup's memory and judgment, it thereby comes to define the category.[39] This phobic escalation in the mechanics of categorization applies 'in all social divisions between "us" and "them," i.e. in all social categorizations in which distinctions are made between the individual's own group and the outgroups'.[40] Research has shown gossip to be an important building-block in this area of social cognition. *All* modes of categorization that reinforce outgroups – not just class-based and religious, but psychiatric too – can be seen as a formalization of gossip. A primary function of gossip is to spot 'free riders', those who contribute nothing to social endeavour but get the same benefits as those who do.[41] Historical evidence supports this – an example being the Nazis's 'useless eaters', the label they applied to the 'feeble-minded' people used as the guinea-pigs for the technology of the Holocaust.[42]

Successfully replicated social psychology experiments have shown that the very act of creating and labelling a category necessarily entails pre-judging it. Even with something as value-free as the relative length of groups of lines drawn on a page, people will judge accurately (i.e. mistakes will be randomly distributed) only as long as the lines remain unlabelled. Call one group of lines A and another B in advance, and preferences will creep in, as well as the exaggeration of differences. All the more so, then, with social categories, which inevitably contain some prior investment of value. Further along the spectrum from prejudice comes stereotyping, says Tajfel (author of those experiments), and at the end, the dehumanization and elimination of the outgroup.[43]

From this it is possible to conclude that inclusion phobia and the concept of intellectual disability are the malignant outgrowth of our adaptive cognitive functioning. Philosophers more generally have written about 'the violence of naming'. The act of labelling an object, the founding gesture of social order, is also the violent imposition of an inherent inequality through language.[44] Any language thus founded (including that of intelligence, and especially its representation as science) is rooted in an arbitrary, irrational act that renders people inherently unequal. So the argument runs. Can we apply this speculation from critical social theory, lacking as usual any joined-up historical specificities, to the concrete pathways which inclusion phobia has taken over the centuries?

Tajfel thought so, or something like it. For him, the dehumanization of others does not just come from an aggregate of individual mind-sets but from a shared ingroup affiliation, and from the relations between it and the outgroup; it is the function of intergroup situations, which are inherently unstable. Hence, he says, facts from history are as relevant, and as verifiable, as facts from experiment.[45] He goes so far as to say that the scientific explanation of social *change* is the core component in building a 'rational model' of social phenomena.[46] As a test case, it will beat the 'blood and guts' examples furnished by sociobiology or evolutionary psychology every time. Adaptive cognitive functioning should be seen as a 'shared psychological process of social change' in which the acceptability of ingroup behaviour towards outgroups undergoes constant transformation.[47] (The prime example once again – both Tajfel's and Gabel's families had been murdered in the Holocaust – is the sudden spike in anti-semitism in the Nazi period and its ensuing downturn.) The categorization process is a continual search not only to establish coherence, but also to maintain it, by always *re*-establishing it anew.

Thus, as well as being rooted in social change, the processes of categorization have a certain structural permanence, in the sense that a 'theory of contents of [outgroup] stereotypes' is possible. 'Where there is dirt there is system', as Douglas also reminds us.[48] Tajfel divides the contents into those characteristics which are already 'assumed to be situational, transitional and flexible, and those which are assumed to be inherent and immutable'. Stereotypes are on the one hand in a continual state of breaking up and reassembling under social pressures, but on the other hand bring order and simplicity to random variation. Thus, although social change will destroy the usefulness of one system of status differentiation, in supplying a replacement it demonstrates the possibility and survival of a *general theory* of how the content of outgroup categories arises, if not of their *actual* content. The common cross-historical thread is the danger they pose: threats to ingroup self-representation and status are formed in new ways at particular historical moments.[49] (Tajfel's work teems with examples, but learning disability is not one of them.)

In his explanation of why ingroup/outgroup characteristics and relationships change Tajfel does not say, simplistically, that the social trumps the individual. Individual histories are intrinsic to socio-historical changes in the ingroup/outgroup dynamic, expressing a general process of socialization. The individual's self-image 'derives from his knowledge of his membership of a social group, together with the value and emotional significance attached to that member-ship'.[50] As we shall see, it is collective self-image and self-esteem alone that constitute what is currently called intelligence – and therefore intellectual disability.

Inclusion phobia: the effectiveness of existing approaches

Along with the authors cited above, I take the pathology to lie in the ingroup and its creation of outgroup categories, rather than in the people thus cate-gorized. Inclusion phobia, because it exists at a deeper cultural level and has a more permanent historical presence than intellectual disability, is the more stable of the two conditions, and is therefore the more appropriate launching-point for research into the other.

Is there a cure? Simply naming it is a start. The theoretical approaches examined above have, as well as some common strengths, some common limitations. Let us start with the latter. The problem is twofold. First, several of the theories that locate the problem within the ingroup and its act of categorizing and labelling others nevertheless belong to that same broad set of mind-sciences whose research has been responsible for the categorizing and labelling in the first place. Not a fatal handicap (after all, the disorder lies only in those subdisciplines that employ concepts of intelligence), but a significant one. Second, they all ignore learning disability. This seems perverse, since within present systems of social organization and status representation, this way of categorizing people is the clearest of all possible illustrations of how an extreme outgroup is created. Clear, that is, as long as one is not stationed behind the pillar of one's own self-esteem.

The two shortcomings are interconnected. Categorization and labelling may lend order to an otherwise chaotic human universe, but as Tajfel himself points out, the fact that they then go on to become stereotypical and therefore *delu-sional* does not prevent the delusions from invading the research community itself.[51] Existing categories, he says, impose a forced choice of definitional criteria on upcoming researchers, imposing some things and ignoring others (nothing illustrates this better than his own failure to mention learning dis-ability). Any discipline that starts out from scientific concepts of subjective intelligence and thus, unavoidably, of an intellectually disabled outgroup, must itself be in some delusionary state. The objective, seemingly neutral rationality of any experiment in the psychology of intelligence becomes no more than a tacit but illicit guarantee of the rationality of the subject doing the experimenting. Psychiatry itself accounts for intellectual disability and anxiety disorder (in our version of it, inclusion phobia) at the same taxonomic level as each other. Yet a scientific discipline that by now undoubtedly classifies as phobic the exclusion of Jews or lepers has the conceptual segregation and (ultimately) elimination of certain 'intellectually' disabled people as the rationale for its own very existence. Intellectual disability is the first condition listed in DSM5. The order is not alphabetical, but no reason is given for the order in which disorders *do* appear. We must assume that pole position is allocated to intellectual disability because on the circuit of normalcy it is the one condition that does not even make the starting grid.

In each of the above theories of outgroup exclusion we could effectively substitute learning disability for some of the illustrations. So why do none of them mention it? Is it just accidental forgetting, or is it because people with learning difficulties (let's say in this case profound or severe ones) do not even qualify as an *out*group, let alone an ingroup? In other words, the people thus labelled do not in the last resort qualify as human. The common view of all the authors is that criteria for categorization are derived from social and cultural contexts. An outgroup for Tajfel can be a group of people you do not identify with (ballroom dancers, golfers), a group you positively wish to avoid being identified with (Essex boys, rednecks), or the one group you would do everything in your power not to be identified with because it would be a matter of life and death (Jews in mid-century Europe). But in addition to these kinds of discrimination, public discussion of which has sparked attitudinal changes over a relatively limited timespan (for example the attainment of political citizenship by women, the European working classes or black Americans), a whole era will also have at its core a largely *unrecognized* but precisely thereby a *primary* outgroup. That is because, historically, the very conceptualization of such an outgroup accounts for the identity of the ingroup. The above authors regard their cited objects of exclusion as temporary victims whose lot in life can be remedied in the medium historical term. What remains invisible is not our core outgroup's existence as such (after all, the label certainly exists) but the fact that actually it is just as much if not more of a historical contingency as those other, secondary outgroups such as women, unskilled labourers or black people. They are secondary in the sense that they have an escape route from their excluded status. And in the recent past the escape route has consisted in being able to show precisely that they are *not* intellectually disabled, do not have lower IQs, and are therefore not like that tiny, genuinely pathological residuum of people over there.

The problem is that learning disability and the people it denotes expose the historically contingent nature of the ingroup itself and its claim to status, threatening not only its social dominance but the means of self-representation ('intelligence') by which that dominance is obtained and maintained. Hence the need to represent the purely psychological elements of the outgroup's identity as a quasi-biological, unchanging natural kind; without that, the ingroup's own status could not be natural or permanent either. That is why learning disability is excluded from the realm of social explanations and theories that have sought to remove the 'natural' label from existing outgroup differences such as race and gender, and why it is absent from the very argument, from outgroup theory as such.

This exclusion from the possibility of argument runs right across the theoretical and political spectrum. If you are a Foucauldian or some other radical social theorist, you may be used to arguing, for example, that psychology is socially constructed, not a hard science like physics or chemistry but a merely human science, or more likely a mere set of power-driven prejudices. In such cases the relationship between observer and observed can easily flip; it is possible to ask who is mad and who is sane within the clinical relationship, or at least to define sanity merely as absence of madness (this is almost routine in current psychiatry). But you have to have a modicum of intelligence in order to do so. Intelligence and intellectual disability, by contrast, form the intergroup relationship that for the present moment cannot be flipped. The presuppositions behind it are absolute.

This becomes clear in the forums where academia and practice meet. There is a fine line between radical critique and disengagement. Policy initiatives may try, for example, to tackle inclusion phobia by closing segregated provisions. Confronted with optimistic social policies like this within an existing regime of power, radical social theorists may often be found in opposition, lined up alongside medical-model positivists in a Coalition of No Tomorrow. What the doctor sees as wild-eyed radicalism the Foucauldian or social constructionist sees as a naïve surrender to neo-liberalism, but their doubt is the same: how can someone disabled in their *intellect* survive in a brutal world? One group is against the possibilities of change because it is conservative and has an urge to protect people, the other because change within any existing regime of power is self-evidently *im*possible. Hence this is a minority that is excluded even from the idea that outgroups can challenge their own marginalization – they are excluded from the ingroup of outgroups, so to speak.

Not only that: they are precisely the outgroup that should be most crucial to the theory, since cognitive ability – attributed first to elite clerical administrators and now to virtually all its subjects – is what convinces the average citizen they have power when they do not. Grant people a specious but quasi-autonomous sphere like this, in the form of meritocratic intelligence or rational consent, and you strengthen their bonds to the power of the state and the markets. Where disability is concerned, to charge governments with neo-liberalism for aiming at paid employment for people with profound learning difficulties (the chance for people with moderate ones would also be a fine thing) is to accept neo-liberalism as an excluding system. It lies within the very definition of such a system to exclude people who can't work or obtain a job through the markets. As Douglas points out, the urge to maintain purity of caste and ingroup cleanliness is rooted in the division of labour.[52] To endorse the idea that people with learning difficulties lie outside a capitalist labour market is thereby to help maintain in its present state the very mechanism you consider to be an excluding one, and thus to endorse the very thing you appear to be challenging. A call for people to have jobs may sound naïve, but demonstrates the possibility of historical change, by challenging the reification mechanisms of a division of labour whose current state is regarded as being as fixed in nature.

The omission of learning disability from these authors' lists of category mistakes and delusions goes hand in hand with their omission of a detailed historical perspective on the particularities of change among outgroups, even the ones they do mention. Restoring the first omission should lead to a restoration of the second, and vice-versa. The creation and exclusion of outgroups may be a collective ingroup disorder, but where the topic is intelligence itself, the word 'collective' indicates not just an ingroup but an ingroup so far in the majority as to be considered a *species*: intelligence is central to the rationality of modern social life, but precisely as such it is also presented as the core natural element in what it is to be human. If the roughly 1 per cent sector of the population with learning difficulties is the primary outgroup of the modern era, then the ingroup is the entire number of those within the band of normal intelligence and above. The distinction between social ingroup (99 per cent) and natural species (100 per cent) having been elided, it is easy to fall for the trick.

The antidote is an awareness of the conceptual history of inclusion phobia. A theoretical account of it has to be something quite different from what Foucault or social constructionism can offer. Although Moore itemizes certain shifts in outgroup patterns, in the last resort he demotes the detailed historical *process* on which such a theory has to be built, in favour of *structure*. His overall picture is largely static, or at best identifies just one big historical landmark. We cannot understand the crucial stage of learning disability in the longer trajectory of inclusion phobia unless we know how it was born or even that it *was* born in the first place, at some point through that trajectory, and how it progressed from its formerly relative status, as at most a secondary aspect of other outgroup categories, to the key role it now occupies as an extreme outgroup among the forms of human self-representation

The importance of that history is therefore, on the one hand, that in terms of actual content extreme outgroups of the distant past have characteristics quite different from today's learning disabled group (thus learning disability is modern), but that, on the other hand, there is a concrete, traceable continuity from one extreme outgroup to the next, from those of the distant past till the present day. What *fuels* that continuity and creates the links in the historical chain, in tandem with the changing material conditions of socio-economic organization, is inclusion phobia. It is in the very acting out of the phobia, and thus in the creation and exclusion of learning disability and the people it denotes, that we build for ourselves what Ludwig Wittgenstein called a 'form of life' distinguishable from that of other animals: that is to say, a species culture (for the moment, one that is centred on the idea of human intelligence). We then jump to a further claim, which Wittgenstein was alert to and which – precisely with regard to 'feeble-minded' people – he refuted: that this culture defines our position in nature.[53]

The fact that learning disability as the characteristic of the core outgroup did not emerge until three centuries ago, and therefore that it may disappear in the future, shows how history can contribute to understanding present-day policies and practices and to acting on them. Gabel calls the ingroup's denial of history 'autistic', but provides little in the way of detail himself, only a broad theory of change as dialectic. Girard provides a greater variety of instances. But both are skewed by their teleological approaches, that is, the prospect of salvation – in Gabel's case Marxist, in Girard's case Christian. Moore too provides detail, but in his case it is skewed by the opposite, dystopian prospect: the inevitable and everlasting grip of institutional power. Tajfel's experiments showing how any act of labelling is intrinsically an attribution of value would probably pass the falsifiability test that signifies an exact science, but they ignore the possibility that learning disability might be their most potent test case.

Leaving aside these criticisms, each of the above approaches supplies invaluable insights that will be applied in what follows. Obsessive-compulsive fears of pollution; morbid rationalism and excess of the identificatory function; schizoid and paranoid thinking; static, 'spatialized' systems for classifying live human relationships; scapegoating and the crisis of differentiation; labelling as inherently value-driven: all these concepts will help us to understand how in the long term, learning disability – the concept, the description, the diagnosis, the corresponding social arrangements – is evidence of a collective disorder. No one can say whether inclusion phobia and its tendency to extremes is characteristic of human societies in general. What we can do is give a detailed account of what has happened to it along the way, to use this as the basis for discerning underlying patterns in the concepts we apply in the learning disability field today, and to think about their future.

Notes

1 Valuing People: A New Strategy for Learning Disability for the Twenty-First Century (2001). London: Department of Health; and Valuing People Now: A New Three-Year Strategy for People with Learning Disabilities (2009). London: Department of Health.

2 R. Hughes et al. (2011) *Journal of Policy and Practice in Intellectual Disabilities* 8 (3), 197–206.

3 Amy R. Krosch and David M. Amodio (2014). 'Economic scarcity alters the perception of race', *Proceedings of the National Academy of Sciences* 111(45), 9079–9084.

4 L. Harris (2006), 'Dehumanizing the lowest of the low: neuroimaging responses to extreme outgroups', in *Psychological Science* 17, 847–853.

5 T. Eagleton (2000). *The Idea of Culture.* Oxford: Blackwell, p. 89.

6 American Psychiatric Association (2013). *Diagnostic and Statistical Manual of Mental Disorders.* 5th edn, Arlington, VA: American Psychiatric Publishing, p. 811.

7 I. Kant (1791/1960). *Religion within the Limits of Reason Alone,* trs Greene and Hudson, Book I. New York: Harper & Row.

8 M. Oliver (1990). *The Politics of Disablement.* Basingstoke: Macmillan.

9 P. Sedgwick (1982). *PsychoPolitics.* New York: HarperCollins.

10 See for example N. Bostrom and A. Sandberg (2009), 'Cognitive enhancement: methods, ethics, regulatory enhancements', *Science and Engineering Ethics* 15, 311–341.

11 S. Rachman (2004). 'Fear of contamination', *Behavior Research and Therapy,* 42(11), 1227–1255.

12 C. Navarrete et al. (2006). 'Disease avoidance and ethnocentrism: the effects of disease vulnerability and disgust sensitivity on intergroup attitudes', *Evolution and Human Behavior* 27(4), 270–82.

13 M. Douglas (1966). *Purity and Danger: An Analysis of Concepts of Pollution and Taboo*, pp. 6, 44, 51.
14 B. Olatunji (2008). 'Core, animal reminder and contamination disgust: three kinds of disgust with distinct personality, behavioral, physiological, and clinical correlates', *Journal of Research in Personality* 42(5), 1243–1259; J. Goldenberg (2001). 'I am not an animal: mortality salience, disgust, and the denial of human creatureliness', *Journal of Experimental Psychology* 130(3), 427–35.
15 P. Rozin et al. (1999). 'The CAD triad hypothesis: a mapping between three moral emotions (contempt, anger, disgust) and three moral codes (community, autonomy, divinity)', *Journal of Personality and Social Psychology* 76, 574–586.
16 L. Harris (2006). 'Dehumanizing the lowest of the low – neuroimaging responses to extreme out-groups', *Psychological Science* 17, 847–853.
17 H. Tajfel (1981). *Human Groups and Social Categories*. Cambridge: Cambridge University Press, p. 39.
18 J. Gabel (1975). *False Consciousness: An Essay on Reification*. Oxford: Blackwell, p. 26. See also *Ideologies* (1997). New Brunswick, NJ: Transaction.
19 R. Girard (1986). *The Scapegoat*. Baltimore, MD: Johns Hopkins University Press.
20 Gabel, *False Consciousness*, p. 43.
21 K. Kosik (1976). *Dialectics of the Concrete: A Study of Problems of Man and World*. Dordrecht: Reidel. pp. 83, 91.
22 T. Stainton (2001). 'Medieval charitable institutions and intellectual impairment c. 1066–1600', *Journal of Developmental Disabilities* 8(2), pp. 19–29.
23 C. Rawcliffe (2006). *Leprosy in Medieval England*. Woodbridge: Boydell Press.
24 M. Jackson (2000). *The Borderland of Imbecility: Medicine, Society and the Fabrication of the Feeble Mind in Later Victorian and Edwardian England*. Manchester: Manchester University Press; G. O'Brien (2013). *Framing the Moron: The Social Construction of Feeble-Mindedness in the American Eugenic Era*. Manchester: Manchester University Press.
25 R. Moore (2007). *The Formation of a Persecutory Society: Authority and Deviance in Western Europe 950–1250*. Oxford: Blackwell, p. vi.
26 Moore, *The Formation*, p. 60.
27 B. Stock (1983). *The Implications of Literacy: Written Language and Models of Interpretation in the Eleventh and Twelfth Centuries*. Princeton, NJ: Princeton University Press.
28 See also I. Metzler (2016). *Fools and Idiots? Intellectual Disability in the Middle Ages*. Manchester: Manchester University Press.
29 Moore, *The Formation*, p. 172.
30 K. Burke (1969). *A Grammar of Motives*. Berkeley: University of California Press.
31 R. Girard (1986). *The Scapegoat*. Baltimore, MD: Johns Hopkins University Press.
32 Girard, *The Scapegoat*, p. 11.
33 Girard, pp. 20, 48, 15.
34 Douglas, *Purity and Danger*, p. 130.
35 Girard, p. 16
36 See Chapter 5.
37 Girard, p. 200.
38 J. Bruner and C. Goodman (1947). 'Value and need as organizing factors in perception', *Journal of Abnormal and Social Psychology* 42, 33–34; Tajfel, *Human Groups*, p. 254.
39 M. Rothbart et al. (1978). 'From individual to group perspectives: availability heuristics in stereotype formation', *Journal of Experimental Social Psychology* 14, p. 237; L. Chapman (1967). 'Illusory correlation in observational report,' *Journal of Verbal Learning and Verbal Behaviour* 6(1), 151–155.
40 Tajfel, *Human Groups*, p. 254.

41 R. Dunbar (2004). 'Gossip in evolutionary perspective', *Review of General Psychology* 8(2), 100.
42 See Chapter 5.
43 Tajfel, *Human Groups*, pp. 40, 141.
44 S. Žižek, cited by M. Withey, *Violence*, in *Bedeutung*, retrieved 21 September 2014.
45 Tajfel, p. 243.
46 Tajfel, p. 128.
47 Tajfel, p. 37.
48 Douglas, p. 44.
49 Tajfel, pp. 132, 139.
50 Tajfel, p. 255.
51 Tajfel, p. 233.
52 Douglas, pp. 34, 128.
53 L.Wittgenstein (1988). *Remarks on the Philosophy of Psychology*. Chicago: University of Chicago Press. Vol. 1, p. 211.

3   Intelligence

We have seen where learning disability stands in relation to inclusion phobia, the more fundamental condition that generates it. Another approach to defining it would be to define what it excludes: intellectual ability, and intelligence. We have not yet said what intelligence is, in precise scientific terms. Physics, for example, has Newton's law of universal gravitation, chemistry Boyle's law of the volume and pressure of gases, and biology Darwin's law of evolution. Does the psychology of intelligence have its own equivalent law, one that governs its existence and provides an equally watertight foundation? What does it say? And who was its author? The empirical evidence from history tells us that the answers are respectively no, nothing, and no one. The definition of intelligence is at best a matter of consensus: not a consensus about the definition of something we know is there, but about whether it is there at all. This must therefore apply likewise to learning disability, since the relationship between the two is polar.

The problem is that consensuses do not last. Consensual means political: a provisional agreement, based not on experimental verification but on the relative authority of whoever is making the definition. The ingroup's essential possession is always up for grabs. With its constant ability to disappear and re-emerge as something entirely other, the concept of intelligence does not belong in the realm of science; it is a classic case of magic, as an anthropologist would describe it.[1] We have already seen how it starts from the relationship of human beings to animals, and from the phobic rituals of domination over them present in all the monotheistic religions.

Intelligence is something we share with animals but perhaps have more of; or it is completely different from animal intelligence; or animals do not have any; or, looking forwards, it is something computers that simulate the human brain (or vice-versa) share with us. From this, just about anything can be extracted by way of definition. For many in the professions it is an individual possession, for the more community-minded it is primarily 'social intelligence'. For behaviourists it is an external descriptor of behaviours, for cognitivists an internal process. For Alfred Binet it is attention span, judgment, critical spirit, and abstraction, for Jean Piaget it is logical reasoning. It has also been information-processing (the acquisition, storing and retrieval of conceptual information);[2] or a general cognitive ability that is also innate;[3] or an ability to modify the structure of one's cognitive functioning in order to adapt to external change;[4] or an assembly of seven discrete items (linguistic, logical-mathematical, spatial, musical, bodily-kinaesthetic, interpersonal, and intrapersonal intelligences);[5] or three (operations, content, products);[6] or a different three (analytic, creative, practical) focused on adaptive behaviour;[7] or four (planning, attention, simultaneous processing and successive processing);[8] or two (practical and creative);[9] or a hundred and eighty.[10] To these we can add problem-solving, forethought, consciousness, communication, and we have barely started. If the reader detects the research-lite hand of Google in some of the above, that is the whole point: the different hits would extend almost infinitely.

Psychologists now tend to deal with this problem of definition liberally. Robert Sternberg, one of the above, admitted that upon asking a couple of dozen authorities for a definition he got a couple of dozen different ones.[11] The American Psychological Association's taskforce, set up precisely to achieve stability on this issue, cited him and added: 'No such conceptualization has yet answered all the important questions and none commands universal assent.'[12] Hence each new piece of research into intelligence must start by a qualifier of the following kind: 'Our working definition of intelligence is essentially that offered by *x*.'[13] In this particular example, *x* had listed 'the ability to reason, plan, solve problems, think abstractly, comprehend complex ideas, learning quickly and learn from experience', ending even more vaguely with '"catching on", "making sense" of things, or "figuring out" what to do'. If a definition offered by *x* (here, the educational psychologist Professor Linda Gottfredson[14]) is valid, why not a definition offered by *y* (myself), or *z* (Jonny)?

The giant research programmes of cognitive genetics consider it legitimate to proceed without clarity, and without even the APA's desire for clarity, about what intelligence is. The idea that definitions of it are relative is familiar enough, but we can easily be fooled by the many ways in which that obvious relativity is finessed. The inviolable importance of a generally accepted concept of intelligence in the modern world leads people to run with the hare and hunt with the hounds. Sternberg himself, for example, explains the problem by paraphrasing the well known 'elephant' story. Three blind men, coming across an elephant for the first time and feeling it all over, each have a different impression: the one feeling its leg says it is like a tree, the one feeling its trunk like a snake, the one feeling its side like a wall. So who is right? Sternberg gives the impression of being about to say that intelligence is therefore a relative concept. But he does not, simply leaving his readers to infer that he has dealt with the problem when he has not. In any case, it is a misrepresentation. The original story said that the blind man thinks the elephant *is* a tree, or a snake, or a wall, not that it is *like* a tree etc. And Sternberg, since he himself offers one of the above definitions, certainly does think it is something.

Any one definition of intelligence will usually be a general heading, comprising several discrete items. The question then arises, what is the boundary separating the items which can be added to intelligence under that definition from those which cannot? If a definition of intelligence can extend from activity *a* to activity *b*, what is there to stop it extending to *c, d, e*, ad infinitum? Answers can only be regressive: that is, the criterion for drawing that boundary can only be 'intelligence', the very concept whose definition begged the question in the first place.[15] In some cases this is accommodated by the addition of an adjective to those aspects that seem not to belong (hence 'emotional intelligence', 'moral intelligence', 'spiritual intelligence', etc.). But this only spins out the original problem. In effect, definitions will coalesce temporarily around a limited number of observable human activities, with no clear boundary between these and other contemporary activities, capabilities or behaviours deemed to lie outside it.

Intelligence and dogmatism

Some of the founders of psychometrics went further and acknowledged the pointlessness of trying to reach a definition.[16] The substance of what it measures is irrelevant. Its scientific basis is predetermined by the fact that it appears to be measurable. Measurability, all on its own, guarantees that it is a real, positive entity. As it can be counted, it can be anything one likes, and most likely a mix of the unexamined presuppositions any particular researcher brings to the table. Nevertheless, the application of psychometrics to research programmes in behavioural and cognitive genetics, which probe the biological causes of intelligence and intellectual disability, has captured the public imagination through the media, where its prestidigitators, backed by large research funds, become spokesmen for a whole society.

It was a century ago that the idea of genetic inheritance was first attached to notions of a 'general' intelligence, or *g* (sporting the same initial as physicists use for gravity). The political stimulus for sharpening up definitions of intelligence was a panic about its deficiencies. In the early twentieth century Charles Spearman, following Francis Galton, was alarmed like his peer elite about the rate of breeding of the unskilled working class and of non-white colonial populations. He injected some statistical sophistication, but the legerdemain remained simple. It went as follows. *Hypothesis*: There is a general intelligence, and if so, the performances of discrete human abilities will correlate. *Method*: Choose certain discrete abilities and measure the performances. *Result*: They correlate. *Conclusion*: There is a general intelligence, and it consists of these discrete abilities.

Spearman's present-day descendants trace the same circle, and the launching-point for research in cognitive and behavioural genetics has, again, been deficiency (this time, mainly language disorder and autism). By no means all of them believe in *g*, the reducibility of all modular abilities to a single measure. But they all assume the existence of intelligence as such, as a scientific object. Its conceptually unstable character doesn't matter, they say, because the heritability rate is generally consistent across every kind of test. Intelligence is whatever intelligence tests measure. What is intelligence? Whatever is measured by intelligence tests. What do these tests measure? Intelligence.

Critics have reduced the biogenetic position to absurdity like this many times, but satire is not enough. As anyone who has had a relationship with a mentally ill person knows, there is no point in directly challenging the logic or veracity of an individual's disordered picture of the world. When the disorder is that of a whole dominant ideology, the far more interesting question is how the exposure of some spurious argument – not just by radical social critics but even by some in the field[17] – is ignored by otherwise sane people. Etiquette in the hard sciences resembles that of duelling. Like calling a gentleman a liar or villain, challenging someone's scientific evidence demands the satisfaction of an immediate response, and this is normally given. Not when intelligence is part of the discussion, however. Critics are not answered but blanked. When the initial sequencing of the human genome led to wild predictions about genetic cures for disorders of the mind, many warned about the political and historical instability of psychiatric categories. In a minor contribution I pointed out, to an audience with an interest in science, the coincidence between the dropping of the 'hysteria' label from DSM and the rise of the feminist movement.[18] Having given the wrong number for the edition in which it had disappeared, I was pursued mercilessly and quite rightly until I confessed my mistake, but my actual challenge, equally a matter of fact, was ignored.

This illustration is not offered by way of complaint but on the contrary to illustrate the absolute *normality* of a non-response. Where the challenge involves something to do with the mind, defendants do not respond or amend as they would if they had made wrong observations of DNA by mistaking base pair CLDN17 for base pair CLDN18. The reason they do not feel obliged is because the issue is not one of biochemical fact in that sense. Yet when the same people announce some DNA-related finding about the causes of intelligence, suddenly it *is* a matter of biochemical fact. This schizoid position must be explained as an endemic disorder of minds suffering from inclusion phobia. The refusal to entertain disconfirmatory evidence is in fact typical of disorders in which there is a paranoid anxiety about some threat, arising in the course of an emotional interaction that enmeshes psychotic processes with pre-existing beliefs ('immigrants all get free housing' is a familiar example).[19] The exact nature of that threat will be discussed in the next chapter.

Existing controversy on the difference between fact and opinion in this field is centred on the opposition between nature and nurture. This controversy is a diversion, however. The current estimate of cognitive geneticists is that heritability and environment each contribute around 50 per cent.[20] This figure looks suspiciously round. Could it just be an artefact, originating from the fact that there are only two items, nature and nurture, to choose from? (The question of why just two, and why *these* two, is dealt with in Chapter 5.) The opposition between nature and nurture seems to reflect a political opposition, between right-wing justifications of social inequality on grounds of unequal intelligence and left-wing optimism about levelling out genetic inheritance with equal educational opportunities. Researchers themselves usually disown any such narrow political allegiances. The presenter of a public radio programme discussing the variability of definitions of intelligence, science communicator and editor of *Nature* Dr Adam Rutherford, claimed that what goes on in the laboratory is unbiased; the politics only starts outside.[21] But the prior question is not just what *goes on* in the lab but what is *present* there in the first place. Intelligence is there, and it is an unstable, already political concept at root.

The issue is not, as the popular science communicators present it, the relationship of DNA to nurture, nor politics of the right–left sort. The weakness in cognitive genetics lies deeper. It is the more basic assumption that the two types of research, into biochemistry and into the mind, can work with each other in the first place. Rutherford defended experimental practice on the grounds that 'When we say that this or that person is clever, we sort of know what we mean.' Now a laboratory normally operates on the basis of what researchers actually do know. Its existence has been verified by scientific method. What they 'sort of' know is another matter. Compressing them into a single aim, to establish biochemical causes of intelligence, is no guarantee that the two realms of knowledge involved are capable of joining up. As the well funded roofer who has tried and failed to mend your leaky guttering will tell you, bonding new plastic to old lead is tricky. If intelligence is a matter of opinion (what we sort of know), no theory that bonds it to DNA (what we do know) is falsifiable. The rules of scientific method do not and cannot apply in this kind of experiment, because there are no conceivable circumstances under which its conclusions can be challenged (again, I do not expect an answer).

Rutherford interviewed another well-known science communicator, Professor Steve Jones, who rightly warned: 'We are entitled to our own opinions, but not to our own facts.' Comparing arguments for the primary influence of nurture with those for the existence of God, he went on to say that 'if somebody has decided to believe something – whatever the evidence – then there is nothing you can do about it' so there is no point even bothering to argue with them, any more than with our notional insane person. Yet what intelligence is, is opinion rather than fact, and in the above case it was the one Jones himself opted to believe in.

This is where history rides to the rescue. Perhaps it is possible to engage with disordered minds after all. The historian R. G. Collingwood is well known for pointing out how important our 'absolute presuppositions' are. For people of any era, certain things were or are beyond question. There has been a prior, unwitting decision to believe. *Absolute* presuppositions are the very ground you are standing on. This is what makes them absolute rather than relative. People do not even find it necessary to propose them as true; to do so could provoke awareness of the possibility that they might not be. To speak about 'sort of' knowing what intelligence is betrays subconscious anxiety about the chasm that might just open up beneath the speaker's feet, especially as it is a presupposition based on ingroup self-esteem.

The historian's task is to explore and reconstruct the past as an outcome of these unquestionable beliefs. We shall examine shortly the absolute presuppositions which existed around status and inclusion phobia in the period immediately before the modern era ('modern' for a historian means roughly the seventeenth century onwards) and the triumph of human reason or intelligence that went with it. The presuppositions of the past may seem entirely obsolete, scarcely capable of being grasped and hence not worth studying. But Collingwood also pointed out that it might be difficult to get round the back of our own without being able to get round the back of them, and vice-versa.[22] Intelligence is an example. Studying the past is useful because it helps us to trace, via gradual, concrete links in a historical chain, the move towards the modern concept of a specifically human intelligence and its elevation into the object of a sacred rite. It also helps us to project into the future, if only to ask at what point this absolute presupposition of our own will have been replaced by something else.

Intelligence and scepticism

All research worth the name starts off by questioning existing knowledge. There is no limit on how deep a question can go. Are the basic categories we currently work with in the field of learning disability a foundation for knowledge, or are they just received opinion?

At the dawn of the modern era, René Descartes made the classic statement of scepticism, which fed into the origins of modern science:

> If someone with a basket of apples was worried that some of them might be rotten and wanted to remove them, so that the rest would not rot too, how would he go about it? Wouldn't he start by emptying the basket completely? Wouldn't he then examine every apple in turn, and put back only the ones he could see were not affected?[23]

The key word is 'completely'. Every item has to be removed for inspection. And for us that includes the very notions of intelligence and learning disability. Do these things really exist, or are they just delusions? We have seen that most research on our topic, sociological as well as psychomedical, ignores Descartes' warning. We take it for granted that intelligence, and therefore intellectual disability and the identity of the people it describes, are sound apples, even if we cannot say convincingly what they are. If the definition of intelligence is exclusively down to consensus and politics, the same must go for its polar opposite. The APA, in setting itself that task of defining intelligence, unwittingly revealed how this works when it excused its failure to do so by saying, 'Scientific research rarely begins with fully agreed definitions, though it may eventually lead to them'. The delusion here is that what goes on in a seminar room and what goes on in a specimen chamber belong in the same class of things.

How does this kind of scepticism contribute to social action? It is not unusual to encounter criticisms of the way the concept is used in practice. Intelligence, and likewise its deficiencies, may seem not to refer to anything real, in the sense of having a permanent existence in nature and an unchanging historical identity, but their conceptual hollowness does not mean we can ignore them. They are the delusions of a whole society and its power structures. Categorizations of our fellow human beings, even if merely verbal, and however illusory they may be, have a direct effect on our lives. Even if categories are only what we want them to mean, they also help to construct exclusive social institutions, spread phobic but apparently normal ways of thinking and doing things, and set criteria for future research and funding. The only way to avoid the normality of exclusion, to negotiate the crevasse in mainstream life, culture and institutions down which some of our fellow human beings vanish, is to set them within a historical and with that a future perspective. It means looking in detail at how specific conceptual categories came to be as they are now, others having been discarded or avoided: by catching them in flight, so to speak. It can help us to intervene effectively in the here and now and in people's future prospects.

If, on the one hand, the long historical perspective shows how ingroup anxieties long ago were about things so entirely different that they bear no relation to a modern concept such as human intelligence, or to the population excluded by it, on the other hand that perspective reveals a continuous trail of categories, a concrete historical totality, within one particular phase of which we find ourselves today. Trawling the historical record we find fruit sound enough to go back in the basket – it just turns out not to be apples.

Particular forms of social organization throw up and require abilities that involve a more or less 'pure' thinking, separable from other human activities. That is not in question. What is in question is people's ideas about what forms and frames its content, and therefore the existence of intelligence as a cross-historical object. Ideas about its historical permanence often take the closed circular form which Gabel regards as typically schizoid. For example, psychology is the study of the mind, yet what we study it with is also the mind. How can one and the same thing be both the thing investigated and the thing that is doing the investigating? In medieval and Renaissance philosophy, the mind was in its ideal state when 'the understanding understands the understanding'. As the philosopher Thomas Hobbes pointed out, this is as absurd as saying that 'sight sees sight', or 'hearing hears hearing'. It collapses in on itself. In what sense were those medieval thinkers doing *psychology*? They were not making everyday case studies of people's minds; they were referring instead to the blessed state of the human soul after death, and to occasional moments of extra-saintly contemplation by themselves. All discussion could be referred back to the operations of divine reason: a transcendent intelligence entirely free from contamination by the body and the senses, which would otherwise distort it.

Modern psychology is nevertheless the direct descendant of medieval philosophy and theology. The circular thinking whereby the investigative tool of a discipline is made of the same stuff as the thing it investigates has material social effects. It acts like a stockade, closing off and protecting the entire knowledge system of an era as it turns its back defensively on any social relationships that might threaten it. This is what Gabel defines as the 'autistic' element in the thinking of a social class or ingroup maintaining its power. Intelligence, as a claim to define the human species, is defending a whole way of life. The notional 1 per cent of people whose character breeds fear of contamination through their association with what lies beyond the purity of the ingroup circle, like the 75 per cent of labouring and money-grubbing masses positioned beyond the medieval elite, evoke the mess and dirt of bodily appetites. As *mere* bodies, they contaminate the sacredness of intelligence.

The medieval thinkers' phobic disgust continues today in transhumanism, a quasi-religious area of study that predicts and aims at ridding ourselves of our corporeal identities. The very word 'transhuman' is in fact an old one. It was first coined by Dante to describe the narrator's state of being when at the end of *The Divine Comedy* he comes to face to face with God. The link to leading present-day transhumanists is not so obscure. Professor Nick Bostrom, a researcher on techniques for discarding bodily influence through cyborgization, continues to cite Anglican bishops in support of this aim, and unwittingly exposes the phobic motives: 'I am apt to think, if we knew what it was to be an angel for one hour, we should return to this world ... with vastly more loathing and reluctance than we would now descend into a loathsome dungeon or sepulchre.'[24] Such ideas are even discussed in the same institutions now as then. The same Oxford University whose medieval theologians once hosted the theory of the immortal soul and its aspiration to a bodiless, angelic state in which communication would took place directly by thought transference, now hosts Professor Bostrom's Future of Humanity Institute, which examines the technical possibilities for 'superintelligence' and the transformation of human beings into pure software that can migrate to other galaxies.

Similarly, the heterodox medieval doctrine of mortalism, which said that the soul dies with the body and only revives and reunites with it at the Day of Judgement, has clear a link forward to cryonics and the MIT neuroscientists' vision of 'uploading' our brains so that they can be scanned and reanimated after death in a computer simulation which, once invented, will be able to resurrect our individual consciousnesses in a matrix where virtual bodies and minds can live forever.[25]

Intelligence and religious delusion

All the definitions of intelligence cited above start with some version of the formula: 'Intelligence is ...' This is an example of what logicians call deductive reasoning: the starting-point is a general premise (in this case, the existence of intelligence), from which logical consequences are drawn. Modern science finds this way of reasoning inadequate. The train of thought that follows, however logical in itself, will be flawed because the premise remains unexamined and therefore can turn out to be a chimera. In the medieval university, where logic was part of the core curriculum, the paradigm case for deductive reasoning was 'God is ...' You presupposed the existence of God, *then* said who he was and why he had to exist. Substitute any psychological category for God, and the same problem will arise by analogy: 'Emotion is ...', 'Imagination is ...', for example. Anyone can complete these predicates with anything they like, having presupposed the prior existence of that category.

'Intelligence is ...', however, is a special case. This is more than an analogy. The God of medieval philosophy *was* Intelligence, by definition. And then, from the late seventeenth century through to the establishment of the modern psychological disciplines, God the Divine Intelligence imperceptibly *became* human intelligence. Our modern category of intelligence is not *like* the concept of God, it *is* the concept of God, by historical derivation. Professor Robert Plomin, currently a major recipient of cognitive genetics funding in the UK, is the direct intellectual descendant of Charles Spearman, the early-twentieth-century inventor of 'general' intelligence, who was the descendant of the leading thirteenth-century theologian St Thomas Aquinas, who in turn was a recipient of divine wisdom. However secular our modern conceptions of what it is to be human may seem, there are certain things we grasp not by analysing but by worshipping them. Intelligence is one. Divine reason has not been secularized, its sanctity has simply been transferred to human beings, as a species.

The notion of an intelligence that is peculiar to humans as a biological species is scarcely three centuries old. It is in fact only one of the many different ways in which we have represented ourselves to ourselves and to each other. During that period, modes of human self-representation changed and competed. In this process intelligence added itself to the stock of prime materials from which ingroup/outgroup categories are made and remade. A succession of individual thinkers has defined it and redefined it as what they themselves possess. In the modern era it has won out, and is now so universal and entrenched that we are incapable of seeing it for what is in essence: namely, a temporary and historically contingent sub-set of the ultimately non-specific claim to be above certain other people. If some individuals do not have more or less of it than others, it cannot exist: hence it is a product of Girard's 'crisis of differentiation'.[26]

And so, finally, we have arrived at the point of definition. Intelligence is a claim to status. To make this absolutely clear: it is not the kind of claim to status that can refer back to some prior, verifiable collateral (like wealth, for example). It is a status claim and nothing else. When we say intelligent we mean better, i.e. better than someone else. The two words are identical and cannot be separated. It is not that if you are more intelligent, you have higher status as a result; nor is it just that the word is loaded with value, as are all terms used to describe human qualities. 'Intelligent' and 'better' are *synonyms*. Intelligence is the act of pulling rank rather than any substantive reason for doing so. No more than that – but also no less, since such abstract claims to status are a formative part of dominant ideologies and social structures, alongside material conditions and in interaction with them, and they have a direct impact on people's lives.

In fact our whole descriptive framework for intelligence and the study of it is a continuation, in pseudo-secular terms, of the medieval view of the cosmos as a hierarchical ladder of nature. At the very top stood divine perfection. All forms of life were by degrees closer to or further off from this perfection which consisted of reason. Our usual perspective is to lump ideas like this with religious or primitive ideas in general, and to contrast them with those of the modern human sciences. Nevertheless, a passage can be traced in concrete detail from thirteenth-century schools of theology to our own futurological institutes, a passage during which there has been no epistemological revolution of the kind that occurred in physics, chemistry or even (despite the best efforts of the evolutionary psychologists) biology, that might call the ladder of nature and its hierarchy of value in question.

The aspiration to cosmic immortality and angelic cyborgization seeks reassurance in concepts of intellectual disability and the possibility of eliminating it. The ladder of nature, still embedded in the psychology of intelligence, tells us that being intellectually disabled marks a lesser degree of perfection. But intelligence is merely the temporary conceptual occupant of a rung that exists *before* any substance or content has been announced. What being intelligent means, once the substance of some specific behaviour or ability has actually entered the discussion, is that this particular ability is of superior value for the era you live in. And so the same goes for the outgroup, which will simply consist of people who are of less value in that specific sense. Even across the present 'cognitive' moment, we have little consensus about what cognition itself consists of; even in the medium term cognitive ability and its correspondingly disabled outgroup are categories as unstable as intelligence itself.

Intelligence and empire

The idea of nature as a hierarchical ladder belongs in a nexus of material social relations. To understand inclusion phobia and ingroup/outgroup formation we have to focus on social history as well as ideas – and more precisely the interpenetration between the two. In the history of religious ideas, the superiority we feel over other animals on the ladder of nature reflects the superiority of some of us feel over other human beings. But that superiority is also embedded in the detailed history of administrative practices. In fact, the conceptualization and possibly the very existence of the most frequently cited components of cognitive ability – information processing, logical reasoning, abstraction – arise directly out of those practices.

The key moment is the rise of empire in the late Roman period, alongside the spread of Christianity. Some preliminaries are necessary, though. Before that, the professional educators of Athens and its mercantile power base, known as Sophists, had already conceived something like an information-processing model which we know about from a drily ironic description of it by Plato. The thinking process in a human being, they said, is like a wax tablet on which impressions are inscribed; some are deeper, some fainter, and thus more or less fit to accommodate, retain or retrieve the information acquired. Some people had deficient mental wax. Deficiency might overlap with lack of legal or political status (slaves, women, non-citizens), but might also be attributed to artisans, who were citizens and had the vote. The overlap between psychological category and social identity was still hazy. In fact even slaves and women belonged in some sense, since the city-state was a society whose model of difference was rooted in integration (each deficient or politically marginalized group had a positive social function) rather than exclusion.

The Greeks are usually thought of as great minds who started us all off down the road of psychology, or as primitives whose naïve ideas we have jettisoned. Mostly they were neither. Nevertheless, that information-processing model does point to some historical continuity from then till now: namely, the assumption that what goes on internally, in the mind, can be described by whatever information technology is around in the external, material world. What features in the discussion of mental and intellectual processes is often just the internalization of something that has a prior existence in the external world. The student listening to a lecture about the mind being a wax tablet would have been scribbling his notes on his personal wax tablet – the writing technology of the time. There is an obvious parallel between saying in 400 BC that the mind is like a wax tablet, in 1200 AD a blank sheet of paper, and in 2000 AD a computer tablet. Greek information-processing theory was a precursor to modern cognitive theory in just this sense: the historical constant is that both are instances of the same techno-fallacy.

Aside from this, we get the first inklings of a specifically modern Western concept of intelligence not from ancient Greece or even the early Roman republic but from the later (Roman) growth of settled empire, from the first century AD onwards, that is. The interaction between social history and the history of ideas becomes clearer with the unprecedented expansion of settled empire and its extraordinary organizational demands. The republic had run a Mediterranean empire of sorts, but its ramshackle political organization and infrastructures were still those of a local city-state. As the system of empire spread, however, the establishment of adequate administrative and legal systems began to sow the seeds of modern bureaucracy. A jurisdiction that stretched from Cairo to Carlisle demanded a universal system of office-holding among locals, to administer property law, taxation, censuses and the rest.[27]

Alongside the introduction of these external controls, people's inner natures and thought processes were also coming gradually under the far-flung scrutiny of Christianity. An orderly system of remote power embedded in local institutions of law and politics required a corresponding form of religion. Here too are some of the important roots of modern intelligence. The idea of the unknown has a social significance everywhere, as Douglas reminds us. In simple societies shamans, and in complex ones priests, to be followed by the mind-sciences, control the distinction between absence and presence, and use this power to deal with contamination. They are in charge of prohibitions and exclusions, acting in support of an unknown, because remote, God, or an unknown, because remote, centre of administration. As this elite 'shuttle[s] back and forth' between the human world and an immaterial, invisible world of the 'spirit' or 'mind' beyond the grasp of ordinary people, its successful exercise of authority hangs on its role as provider of solutions to problems arising in social arrangements.[28]

'Prohibitions', says Douglas 'trace [both] the cosmic order and the ideal social order'. Exclusions too, we might add. Christianity's practical means for the systemization and supervision of people's inner, intellectual natures took the form of the catechism. Early on, the people tested by this kind of baseline assessment would have been mainly apprentice theologians, at a fairly high level (not local priests, for example, who tended to be illiterate). They were very few, but they would also be the ones who, if found deficient, would contaminate the purity of the ecclesiastical elite and its institutions, and whom it was therefore crucial to exclude.

What were the core ideas in which these apprentices were trained? During the third century AD two seminal ideas about the mind, associated with two key figures, arose: (1) the establishment of Intelligence or (depending on context) Intellect as a general, overarching entity; and (2) the definition of man as a 'rational animal'.

The first of these was due to school of thought headed by a philosopher named Plotinus, who had absorbed and radically altered Greek thought in this field. He uncoupled the realm of the unknown from local deities and recreated it on a grand unitary scale. For a Roman imperial administration espousing Christianity, that realm now consisted of the Divine Intellect, in its supreme self-contemplating state. Plotinus transmitted this idea on to the medieval knowledge systems, via the Arab philosophers; the modern concept of a general intelligence is a long-term historical descendant of his unashamedly circular theory. Of course the concept of intelligence *per se* underwent many transformations in the centuries in between. It is above all in methods of exclusion that we find the stable historical perspective in which to set it.

The second seminal idea came from a student of Plotinus named Porphyry, who coined the formula 'Man is a rational animal.' In doing so, he took a major step on the path towards the modern cognitive concept of man, pinpointing human beings on the ladder of nature at an overlapping mid-point between the animal realm and divine reason. His ubiquitous phrase became the founding principle of medieval cosmology, and subsequently of what we now call the human sciences. It was the focal point of a system for the organization of knowledge, including knowledge about human beings, that would last.

If the shaman's method is to mediate between the unknown and the here and now, as a way of fixing social problems, in a complex imperial society it had to be adjusted to the extended character of that society's rule. Ways of describing and categorizing people, while remaining in touch with the mystical and spirit world, had to be made more systematic as social and political relations became more stretched, geographically and commercially. It should come as no surprise, then, to find that Plotinus and Porphyry, both hardcore mystics, were also personal friends of highly pragmatic emperors. The sixth-century writer Boethius, to whom medieval Europe owed its knowledge of Porphyry's formula, had been a Roman consul. The idea that intelligence marked the place of human beings in the distribution of natural species was thus a political principle before it became a psychological one. No wonder man was a rational animal, when the people responsible for organizing this place for him in a system of natural categories were those at the centre of power, responsible for organizing the extended social relations of empire's outreach and for bringing remote populations into line.

Intelligence and bureaucracy

Nevertheless, in this formula reason still overlapped with the divine intellect, and was accessed only secondarily by human beings. Once the late medieval structures of imperial, ecclesiastical and legal administration required a professional clerical caste, only then could the idea begin to grow of a specifically *human* reasoning that had a separate, objective, observable existence and a tightly classifiable place in the natural world. The people who modelled it were, of course, that caste. Information-processing, logical reasoning and abstraction: these were bureaucratic organizational procedures out there in the external world first; only subsequently did one social group start to internalize these things in the subjective picture it had of itself, and from there to think of them as skills characteristic of the human species.

The need to file things in the external, material world leads to the idea of filing internal mental ones ('abstraction'); the magic circle of intelligence and its ingroup is then sealed when that internalized process is itself re-externalized, as an objective fact of psychology. This illustrates the broader process within the mind sciences in general by which thinghood is attributed to the invisible, intangible qualities of human relationships; pre-existing objective structures are identified and located within the human individual by a process of metaphorical extension, and once that is done they are reified as 'psychological objects'.[29]

When theologians and philosophers in the first universities maintained that information-processing and the rest were archetypally human, they meant *they themselves* were the archetypal humans, as did their ex-students embarking on careers in administration and the professions. The latter, finding themselves in a social hierarchy that had been founded on military skill and whose corresponding internal quality was honour, launched the process in which the key internal quality came to be the new human reason instead; centuries later, these people have expanded to become a caste to which everyone – or almost everyone – belongs.

The caste was rooted in material interests. Roman-style remote administration was continued by the empires around the Mediterranean that followed, then became tighter and more unified through the system of extended landholding we call feudalism. A patrilineal system of inheritance came to predominate. The clerical caste's position within the elite was subordinate because their elder brothers inherited the land and thus also the primary internal and personal attributes of honour and bloodline. Some clerks' paternity made their own status honourable too, albeit less so, and this ruled out dishonourable alternative careers such as trade or banking (that is, in theory – actual social history is another matter and there was plenty of social mixing). It was therefore all the more urgent for them to pursue their own characteristic status claim. The first church fathers had not boasted about how clever they were. But skilled, literate administrators and other professionals created a human intellect in their own image to place at the centre of the natural world, because it offered them the capture, by alternative means, of a status initially barred to them. It also gave many of them the chance to benefit from the internationalization of trade sparked by the Crusades, which demanded their skills as it increased the power of ambient wealth and capitalist enterprise in proportion to landholding. In this alliance between self-interest and self-esteem, everyday cleverness was ascending the scale of value, with serious consequences for those who were unclever in such matters.

The nobility, itself not always very ancient, saw the rising clerical and professional class as upstarts, threatening its own position which it had come to regard as natural. Literacy and numeracy, rather than honour, became the route to power for people whose birth had denied it to them. Clerks with pens replaced enforcers with swords as the local agents of government, as it became more unified and replaced oral procedures with written ones. As Moore puts it, the professionalization of government created a 'rival system of loyalties and values'.[30] However, that is not entirely how the history of status and self-representation works. Once these professionals, joined now by people of even humbler origin, acquired landed estates or a title, they were quite happy to spout their own lines about honour and genealogy. These lines became more emphatic, not less, as the modern era approached. That, and not just a fashion for the classics, was why jobbing lawyers in the eighteenth century sat for their portraits dressed as Julius Caesar. They even claimed descent from him by blood. It is true, as Moore continues, that they also had 'above all their own flag – reason – in whose name they claimed to rule'. But in their minds, their reason melded with their honour, and vice-versa. That was how ingroup status was expanded but also refurbished with a new kind of halo, and outgroup status reassigned accordingly.

Abstraction and logical reasoning: historical contingencies

Psychology as a distinct discipline has promoted abstraction and logical reasoning as the archetypal abilities of the human subject. Their first formal description coincides with the founding of the first universities around 1200, and it was from them too that the idea of human intelligence as a species marker began to emerge. For our purposes here we can treat the various terms – intelligence, intellect, reason, understanding – as interchangeable, even if at the time their meanings were distinct. According to the leading medieval thinkers no mere human can access divine reason because the soul – broadly what we mean today by the mind – has not only a rational part but a 'sensitive' part too, i.e. tied to the senses and bodily appetites. Original sin meant that the latter always prevail, so that our need to rely for knowledge on our external bodily senses means that any intellectual abilities that are *merely* human are corrupted by their interactions with the world of matter. Some thinkers drove in the thin end of a wedge here, claiming that a mortal philosopher at the top of his game might just occasionally be able to hook up with the divine intellect. By the nineteenth century this kind of optimism had prevailed, and the divinity of the rational soul, now dressed up as something entirely secular, was finally attributed to the human species as a whole.

Abstraction, at this time, meant sorting the particular into the general by selecting what various things have in common. Particular *objects*, perceived by the senses, could be allocated to discrete conceptual categories, known as universals – a way of sorting sameness and difference. A moment's thought will tell us that the categories into which we sort inanimate objects, let alone human beings, arise through cultural and historical serendipity. We have ready quips such as 'Intelligence is knowing a tomato is a fruit, wisdom is knowing not to put one in a fruit salad.' In non-Western cultures too, modern systems of categorization can likewise get subverted.[31]

Anthropologists are especially fond of just-so stories about distant peoples who classify things differently from the way modern societies do. Relativism of this sort, however, does not fully answer doubts about the ontological status of abstraction. The history of inclusion phobia allows for a more effective critique. The Greeks had been fond of creating abstract nouns out of ordinary ones (e.g. *politeia*, 'polity' or 'form of government', out of *polis*, 'city'). However, they had no abstract noun that meant 'abstraction'. It was only the medieval philosophers who came up with a dedicated term. Reflecting the clerical administrator's day job at a higher intellectual level, abstraction has subsequently become ever more important to the psychology of intelligence, which sees 'same and different' as the root of cognition. One glance at current forms of assessment such as WISC tests will show how refined the notion of abstraction has since become. Its historical context shows that it started out as a disparate array of things. It was born as and subliminally remains, all at once: (a) the sorting of particular instances under general headings; (b) the 'abstraction' (in the sense of separation) of divine intellect, or today a perfectible general intelligence, from the world of matter; but above all (c) a practical means of categorizing people, often for the purposes of control and decontamination.

As for logical reasoning, this too is usually seen as starting with the Greeks. But with them, logic was an objective system for the construction of arguments. That was all. They had no precise concept of some corresponding logic that might be going on within the individual mind. It was the late middle ages, rather, when logical reasoning became seen as a process within the human subject. And the human subject then became itself an object of that subject's own study, thus closing the circle we now take for granted. Moreover the definition of 'man', as in 'man is a rational animal', became the paradigmatic illustration of objective logical procedure, from which other illustrations were derived. Textbooks on logic in general usually began with that particular illustration. From the sixteenth century this ersatz logic, spuriously attributed to Aristotle, formed the backbone of the proliferating genre of professional manuals for people working in law, medicine and the church.

The main purpose of its apparently neutral principles was to give scientific credence to their own expertise and status, and the idea of a logical reasoning within the individual is now one of the absolute presuppositions of the human sciences. Piaget termed it 'mental logic'. The rigorous flavour of the phrase seems to confirm as scientific his own arbitrary description of what this supreme human ability is.[32] More recently, there is 'mental logic theory', which considers cognition as a 'machine'.[33] Such descriptions of what is to be human remain ways of locating the species on the medieval ladder of nature. Historically, the idea of mental logic as a possession of the individual mind arose jointly with the social aspirations of the people claiming to have it.

From the elite world of that original professional and clerical caste, it too has now become the property of 'everyone'. Again, this may seem to make the history too elastic. True, between the twelfth and twenty-first centuries there has been a total transformation of the content and methods of logic considered as an objective, self-standing system; the medieval syllogism has given way to modern mathematical and symbolic logic. But there is also continuity. Common to the twelfth and twenty-first centuries is the idea of logic as the subject, object and method, all at once, of the psychology of cognition. Several hundred years ago, this blancmange started to be the jus-tification for deciding what is and is not reasonable in the everyday practices of law, religion, medicine, and eventually of the classification of human cognitive and behavioural types.

Intelligence and the consecration of status

The elements of social history I have referred to so far are connected to high-level discussion about how human beings fit within the cosmological frame of nature. Coming down to earth a little, how did intelligence start to play such a central role in the everyday ways people have of representing themselves to each other?

The existence of a specifically human intelligence was of course recognized outside the sanctified world of the social, educational and religious elites. Cleverness and wit of some sort were crucial to the rapidly increasing division of labour and expansion of trade.[34] However, this sort of quality had at first none of the divine overtones that the philosophers' 'reason' and 'intelligence' had. Nor could it. If it had, some of that sacredness would have rubbed off on to its plebeian possessors, and that would have devalued the aspirational caste above them. The everyday wit required for business transactions or manual occupations had a negative profile in those higher echelons. The many self-help gurus of the time, who penned conduct manuals for the elite and especially its new arrivals, dismissed it as low cunning, where 'low' was both a social and a moral judgment on precisely the skills those new arrivals had exercised in order to ascend. Meanwhile, in religion, everyday reasoning was positively harmful, to be ejected from the mind of anyone trying to contemplate divinity or, as the Reformation demanded, to communicate personally with God. In such contexts it was a pollutant.

At a certain point it began to transcend its vulgar and profane origins. This sacralization of everyday wit was also the secularization of divine reason. They intertwine, are part of a single process, from the late sixteenth century onwards, with a particularly sharp turn at the end of the seventeenth. More and more, everyday abilities could bestow you with social merit; thus they were becoming sanctified in their own right, at the same time as the higher-level concept of 'intelligence' to which they increasingly contributed was being relocated to the secular realm of the sciences.

To explain this history in a little more detail, we need some structural framework. I have said above that intelligence is a claim to status *as such*, not to the kind of status that refers to some verifiable object with a prior and separate existence. In this sense it is like celebrity. Just as some celebrities are famous for being famous, the ingroup is intelligent by virtue of its intelligence. Rather than offering concrete collateral for status, it is what I have explained in detail elsewhere as a *mode* of status: a channelling process, through which certain arbitrarily chosen characteristics or abilities become a supreme abstract quality demanding worship from others.[35] The halo is so dazzling as to prevent looking at it long enough to see what it is made of, if anything.

There have been other such modes, aside from intelligence. During the sixteenth and early seventeenth centuries, the chief status icons were grace (religious) and honour (secular). Gradually, wit and a specifically human intelligence started to compete with them ideologically, while at a deeper level collaborating with them to maintain and/or restructure social hierarchies. Most readers of this book would not think of honour or grace as objects belonging to the same class of things as intelligence, but as superstitions or at best obsolete curiosities. Although their presence is still acknowledged in certain cultures (Hispanic or South Asian in the first case, religious sects in the second), they are rarely seen as quantifiable and measurable properties of the mind, in the way we regard intelligence. Yet they were seen that way four or five centuries ago, when they dominated Western European cultures. Moreover, they had that same 'modal' social function, mediating between the realm of some real concrete collateral or social power and that of status as a purely abstract goal.

In the case of honour elites, the collateral was possession of ancestral land. Accordingly, honour was also a component part of your soul or mind, a reified internalization of the landed estate. It was fixed, and thus predetermined, by the quality of certain natural particles in your blood (a notion successfully cited in the British courts as recently as the 1960s, when a hereditary peer first tried to renounce his title). If it was confirmed and certified by your possession of a title, it was also empirically verifiable by a science known as Blazon. True, there was a passing nod to the idea that the odd commoner might cultivate enough 'virtue' to earn himself a title, as long as he topped this up with services to the state or flat cash. Honour, as the sign of gentle status, guaranteed your biological separation from that large outgroup of the plebeian rabble. Being a gentleman entitled you to rule; in your group privilege of 'magistracy' lay the good of the commonwealth as a whole. Honour was as real a category as intelligence, and indeed partly encompassed it. If you were born a gentleman, your honourable station just *was* your superior intellect: the word ability denoted, indiscriminately, both intellectual prowess and possession of land (the Latin word *potentia* covered both). They were a single concept, and to lack one kind of ability was to lack the other.

Status was also a matter of local social histories, between whose cracks conceptual history tends to sprout. The sanctification of intelligence grew from sixteenth- and seventeenth-century social processes whose roots lay in the centralizing tendencies of the absolute state, as it sought the aura of respect necessary for its self-protection. This had once been obtained from popular acclaim for exemplary rulers and only lasted as long as living memory; now it was available through the approbation of the literate professional who could record and thus preserve the ruling class' legitimations of its own power.

In religious contexts, elites saw themselves as superior because they possessed grace. This was an inner ability that was also predetermined by God, and likewise restricted to a small distinct group. It was fixed in your biological nature, 'seminally' (i.e. at conception or before), with a passing nod to the idea that some people – Bunyan's Pilgrim, for example – might be able to work at acquiring it. In theory, grace guaranteed your elite status in this life and salvation in the next, as one of the 'elect'. It separated you from the surrounding outgroup, the herd of hell-bound 'reprobates'. In seventeenth-century England it entitled you to membership of a 'rule of the saints' by which you could lay down the law on other people's behaviour, for their own good. Grace was as real as honour or intelligence. Moreover, you could usually assume that elect status was passed on to your children, like a hereditary title. It consisted of three things: regeneration (becoming a new man), justification (having this confirmed by divine law) and sanctification (the ability to sustain it). The first two were instantaneous and imposed from without by God. Sanctification, however – we shall come across it again – was a gradual process and came from within, from your own efforts once you were regenerated. Hence it was also called 'habitual grace'. Although in theory it was hubristic to seek to know who (including yourself) was elect and who not, it was a proxy sign that could be assessed on a regular basis by having the priest question you on your catechism.

The papacy sought power to prescribe memory, as a way of preserving itself and projecting its line of authority into the future; it did so by replacing local communities' informal elevation of a few extra-holy individuals with the official process of canonization. (Likewise when the cult of relics disappeared, it was not because reason had triumphed over superstition but because of the intellectual centre's distaste for any grass-roots claim to authenticity that came from unlearned 'idiots', local custom, or the geographical margins.[36]) Protestantism subsequently located sainthood within elect individuals. Their state of preparation for grace would in the eighteenth century become a reasoned faith, which in turn has since become secular reason *per se*, distributed among a meritocratic mass of reasoning individuals.

Modern meritocratic elites, likewise, are superior because they possess intelligence. Once more, this is a predetermined inner ability. It too is fixed 'seminally' (this time of the genetic type) – with a passing nod again to nurture and personal effort. Intelligence gives you social status, separating your DNA from that of the common herd who don't make the grades because they are not naturally equipped for upward mobility. It entitles you, as a somebody with more of it, to talk first (and down) to run-of-the-mill nobodies with less or none of it. And few of us would challenge the general consensus that requiring intellectual ability from people who run things is for the good of society. Intelligence appears to be a real category, just as honour and grace did to our sixteenth-century forebears, because like them it is measurable. We shall see in Chapter 7 the precise forms in which these latter were 'scientifically' assessed.

This historical evolution enables us to see how the claim to natural intellectual ability and the claim to social status are identical. It's not that a claim to social superiority can be used to support a spurious claim to intellectual superiority, or vice-versa. A claim to one just *is* a claim to the other. Modern, intelligence-based meritocracy is a passing contortion in the spectacular historical circus of posturings about status. As quaint in its way as grace and honour, the thing we call intelligence reveals itself to be a self-referential bid for status and that is all.

On a long historical view, intelligence is no more a biological or natural kind, and cognitive science no less a pseudo-science, than grace or honour. The difference between past elites and today's rule by exam-passers is not between less and more social mobility, rooted in natural and thus justifiable distinctions, but between alternative expressions of a single purpose: closing off privilege. And if today's meritocrat is the new aristocrat, yesterday's aristocrat was the old meritocrat. Tudor gentry, heraldically assessed and certified, were still anxious to cultivate book learning as well, if only because most could not trace their bloodline back more than a few decades. They started to cultivate virtue, and intellectual virtue in particular, only once they became alarmed by the sudden spike in social mobility around them. Too many 'new men' (the dismissive phrase of the period) were being granted coats of arms by his/her gracious majesty, in return for professional assistance or a gratuity. As for the religious elite, that phrase 'new man' had an entirely different connotation: it meant being born again. But this elite too, like the supposedly old nobility, were under the threat of being swamped. The Book of Revelation's estimate of 144,000 elect could not accommodate the aspirational influx of all those who, thrust upwards by the rapid spread of literate Bible study, began to suspect they too were in grace.

The victorious emergence of intelligence from the other two modes went with cultural changes that saw professional merit and its diffusion across increasing social strata begin to usurp or merge with that of elect status and of rule by hereditary line. The most radical early ideas about political democracy dovetailed with the idea that grace might extend to all, not just the elect. During the English Revolution of the mid-seventeenth century one of its outstanding figures, Gerrard Winstanley, a socialist and an advocate of universal suffrage as well as a religious visionary, consciously substituted the word Reason wherever his readers would expect to find the word God. 'The spirit of the Father is pure Reason' he says, and 'therefore man is called a rational creature' because God dwells in every creature and 'supremely in man'.[37] But Reason here is not a metonym for God. When Winstanley says 'Reason is the King of righteousness' he means it literally, like the French revolutionaries who would set up altars to Reason a century later. In making a point of this substitution, he is anticipating something far more characteristically modern: that the common factor in definitions of intelligence which extend to 'everyone' is not its secular, everyday character but its sacredness.

The ingroup created out of intelligence went further than its predecessor groups in establishing an extraordinarily wide base, where its social definition was now aligned with that of the natural species. The outgroup, correspondingly, has reduced in size to the point of sheer pathology. Its species membership is no longer questioned rhetorically, like the sixteenth-century 'multitude' constantly described as bestial by its superiors, but scientifically, via the new, statistically based concept of the abnormal.[38] When 'idiot' had meant a lay person – neither owning land nor professionally initiated in law, medicine or the church, but clever enough (or not) to make their way in the world – its pathological sense only applied to members of the elite who were incompetent to manage their estates. Meanwhile honour and grace entailed specific outgroups of their own, whose dangerous contaminating potential meant they had to be weeded out by assessment: people without ancestry in the first case, and reprobates predestined for hell, in the second. Negative types were thus plentiful – the majority of the population, in fact. If intelligence belongs to the same conceptual category as honour and grace and sprang out of them and from the competition between them, the same holds true for their respective outgroups, as we shall now see.

Notes

1 M. Mauss (1972). *A General Theory of Magic*, translated by Robert Brain. London: Routledge.
2 U. Neisser (1967). *Cognitive Psychology.* New York: Appleton-Century-Crofts.
3 C. Spearman (1950). *Human Ability.* London: Macmillan.

4 R. Feuerstein (1990). 'The theory of structural modifiability', in B. Presseisen (ed.), *Learning and Thinking Styles: Classroom Interaction*. Washington, DC: National Education Associations.

5 H. Gardner (2011). *Frames of Mind: The Theory of Multiple Intelligences*. New York: Basic Books.

6 J. Guilford (1967). *The Nature of Human Intelligence*. New York: McGraw-Hill.

7 R. Sternberg (1985). *Beyond IQ: A Triarchic Theory of Intelligence*. Cambridge: Cambridge University Press.

8 J. Das et al. (1994). *Assessment of Cognitive Processes*. Needham Heights, MA: Allyn & Bacon.

9 R. Sternberg (1997). *Successful Intelligence: How Practical and Creative Intelligence Determine Success in Life*. New York: Penguin Putnam.

10 J. Guilford (1988). 'Some changes in the structure of intellect model', *Educational and Psychological Measurement* 48, 1–4.

11 R. Sternberg and D. Detterman (1986). *What Is Intelligence? Contemporary Viewpoints on Its Nature and Definition*. Norwood, NJ: Ablex.

12 U. Neisser et al. (1996). 'Intelligence: knowns and unknowns'. *American Psychologist* 51 (2), 77.

13 R. Nisbett (2013). 'Schooling makes you smarter: what teachers need to know about IQ', *American Educator* Spring, 10–39.

14 L. Gottfredson (1997). 'Mainstream science on intelligence: an editorial with 52 signatories, history, and bibliography', *Intelligence* 24(1), 13–23.

15 K. Danziger (1997). *Naming the Mind: How Psychology Found Its Language*. London: Sage, pp. 66ff.

16 See for example A. Binet (1905). 'Méthodes nouvelles pour le diagnostic du niveau intellectuel des anormaux', *L'année psychologique* 11, 191. T. Kelley (1929). *Scientific Method*. Ohio: Ohio State University Press.

17 See for example J. Michell (1999). *Measurement in Psychology: A Critical History of a Methodological Concept*. Cambridge: Cambridge University Press.

18 C. Goodey, 'Genes that are all in the mind', *New Scientist*, 7 June 1997.

19 D. Freeman et al. (2002). 'A cognitive model of persecutory delusions', *British Journal of Clinical Psychology* 41, 331–347.

20 R. Plomin et al. (2012). *Behavioral Genetics*. 6th edn. London: Worth Publishers.

21 *Intelligence: Born Smart, Born Equal, Born Different*, aired 6 May 2014, BBC Radio 4.

22 R. Collingwood (2005). *The Idea of History*. Revised edn. Oxford: Oxford University Press.

23 R. Descartes (1983). *Oeuvres*, vol. 7. Paris: Vrin.

24 G. Berkeley (1732/1948). *Alciphron: or the Minute Philosopher*, in A. Luce (ed.), *The Works of George Berkeley*. London: Nelson, p. 172, cited in N. Bostrom (2008), 'Why I want to be a posthuman when I grow up', in B. Gordijn and R. Chadwick (eds), *Medical Enhancement and Postumanity*. Berlin: Springer.

25 S. Seung (2012). *Connectome: How the Brain's Wiring Makes Us Who We Are*. New York: Houghton Mifflin, pp. 233ff.

26 See Chapter 2.

27 C. Ando (2000). *Imperial Ideology and Provincial Loyalty in the Roman Empire*. Los Angeles: University of California Press.

28 Douglas, *Purity and Danger*, p. 90.

29 K. Danziger (1990). *Constructing the Subject: Historical Origins of Psychological Research*. Cambridge: Cambridge University Press.

30 Moore, *The Formation*, p. 130.

31 See for example R. Keller (2007). *Colonial Madness: Psychiatry in French North Africa*. Chicago: University of Chicago Press.

32 J. Piaget with B. Inhelder (1958). *The Growth of Logical Thinking from Childhood to Adolescence*. New York: Basic Books.
33 M. Braine and D. O'Brien (eds) (1998). *Mental Logic*. Mahwah, NJ: Lawrence Erlbaum.
34 A. Murray (1978). *Reason and Society in the Middle Ages*. Oxford: Oxford University Press.
35 C. Goodey (2011). *A History of Intelligence*, ch. 5.
36 Stock, *The Implications of Literacy*, p. 244.
37 G. Winstanley (1648). 'Truth lifting up its head among scandals', in G.Sabine (ed.) (1948), *The Works of Gerrard Winstanley*. New York: Russell and Russell, p. 110.
38 See Chapter 7.

4   Difference

Inclusion phobia creates an abstract template of difference, whose specific outgroup occupants periodically change and are reinvented. This chapter is about how learning disability has come to fit the template. The fact that we started with intelligence and are only now moving on to the outgroup is not because we are following normal textbook procedure, in which intelligence is a given and learning disability, as the absence of it, trails along behind.[1] That would be to fall in with the intelligent ingroup's view of itself as a natural species, from which exceptions to the rule derive. Here, the purpose of putting intelligence first was entirely different. It was to demonstrate that the concept of intelligence too is a primary product of inclusion phobia.

In fact the sequence often runs *from* disability *to* intelligence. Here, for example, is Douglas Detterman, co-author of the 'two dozen definitions' questionnaire, on the difficulty of defining intelligence:

> Words like moron, idiot and imbecile all started off as scientific terms, but they've been corrupted by common use … So I think a better approach is to define things like general intelligence, or *g*, where we have a mathematical definition, and where we can attempt to get a scientific explanation of the construct.[2]

The 'obviously' scientific status of the former is the trigger for reconstituting that of the latter. This is true even at a precise and detailed level, as we shall see: the designation of new outgroup characteristics leads to a refashioning of the ingroup. Each of its status claims is etched in place by the existence of its respective outgroup; they give the illusion of substantive, determinate and permanent form to what is, albeit in the long term, transient. In the case of bodily disease, historians of medicine have noted how routinely the pathological determines the normal.[3] So much the more, then, in the case of intellectual states, where the pathological characteristics can be arbitrary. At the very least, the notions of intellectual ability and disability are binary but co-dependent opposites, holding each other up in a static abstraction typical of dominant ideologies: a form of 'splitting' that would qualify for Gabel's description of ideology as schizoid. In so doing they form the ultimate kind of *difference*.

There is of course another way of looking at difference. We could celebrate it, as diversity. This seems radical and enlightened: a central principle of today's liberal democracies is that difference is persecuted, and that this situation should be remedied. Black/white, straight/gay, male/female binaries should become two-way streets, transcending inequality and discrimination. But the notion of diversity is actually no more than an abstract expression of liberal democracy's status quo, whose basis lies in competence and rational consent. All social systems accommodate difference in some way, because all social systems can only function through the existence of more than one group – even if relationships between them are unequal because some groups are situated at the margins. But the kind of difference that qualifies someone for membership of an *extreme* outgroup, and thus as the target of inclusion phobia, is not some inequality within a whole system but a difference that by definition lies outside it.

Girard explains this through scapegoating theory. The scapegoated group – whatever features may constitute it at a particular point in history – is the product, he says, of the structural crisis created by an impending *lack* of difference within a social system. The threat represented by the intrusion of an extreme outgroup into the system, says Girard, is that the latter might then 'differ from its own difference', i.e. not contain any difference at all – in which case it would cease to exist as a system.[4] The present system, however, is surely the meritocratic one whose rationale and very existence is constituted by intelligence and a reasoning autonomy. What does *this* social and conceptual system exclude? Obviously learning disability, but Girard does not mention it. Instead, he gets into a complicated analogy about physical disability instead. The human body is a whole system of anatomical differences and usually, he says, we do not see that as a problem, whereas difference as physical disability is 'terrifying'. It seems to threaten the entire system by 'disturbing the differences that surround it'. It 'reveals ... the system['s] relativity, its fragility, and its mortality': not an alternative norm, but abnormality.

Now it is true that the exclusion of people with physical disabilities is typical of a mainstream culture such as our own that reacts obsessively against bodily impairments and their intimations of mortality. But an external constraint such as the built environment does not allocate to that individual an inferior place on the ladder of nature, at least not directly. Yes, social structures are *like* anatomical, physical structures, but with learning disability Girard could have got the real thing. We see here how the extreme outgroup, lying by definition outside a whole system (in our own case, the intelligence society), remains largely unacknowledged even within existing theories of exclusion, let alone in the dominant ideology's sermons about diversity. As for learning disability's own radical advocates and activists, the difficulty of seeing inclusion phobia as the primary disorder, or of seeing a prospect for doing anything about it, sucks many of them too into those same anodyne liberal pieties. For people with learning difficulties (as currently defined), neither orthodox political pluralism nor radical relativism is a level playing field.

The difference targeted by inclusion phobia in its present state is focused on the mind. This, unlike bodily difference, is invisible, which means it is a prime source for magic and shamanism. The concrete make-up of this invisible realm is a series of internalizations of external phenomena, as we saw above for intelligence. Two examples of this kind of conceptual prestidigitation will suffice, both drawn from the field of education.

One is the classification of learning disability as a special educational need. In social policy, the idea of needs surfaced in the concepts and practices of the post-war welfare state, and drew partly on Victorian philanthropy. It referred to constraints on a person's life that were largely external and beyond their control, the chief example being poverty. William Beveridge's term for such externalities, however, had been 'evils'. Here we get a whiff of the essentially religious origins of utilitarianism, rooted as it originally was in fear of the Devil.[5] 'Needs' was the politicians' substitute term. It has transferred the implicitly negative value from those external social structures to the internal realm of the individual child, subjectivizing it as a poverty of the inner person. When a school says, as it so often does when pronouncing on diversity, 'We believe in inclusion as long as we can meet the child's needs', it certainly sounds better than 'as long as they are not evil'. It is nevertheless an excluding formula because it opens up the possibility of an ultimate or extreme outsider whose needs cannot be met: not just an excluding system but a system that necessarily *creates* exclusion through the creation of an entirely negative identity.

A second example is 'barriers'. This term originally entered education through the literature on inclusive schooling, which coined the phrase 'barriers to inclusion' to denote the obstacles thrown up by excluding systems.[6] It did not take long for the UK Department of Education, having in the interim accepted the surface language of inclusion, to be routinely using the phrase 'barriers to learning' to denote an internal feature of the child. Where possible, such barriers are to be overcome (cured) by pedagogical intervention. Tacitly, then, this still marks out a separate conceptual and of course geographical space for incurables, whose internal barriers are not capable of being overcome.

Ability and disability: chicken or egg?

Exclusion on intellectual grounds always appears to be after the event, as if it were the inevitable response to some natural disaster. Yet the educational, clinical and developmental psychologies that underpin it are not some permanent objective science that one day turned its hand to excluding people: their very coming into being was *result* of a prior urge to exclude. In historical perspective, the causal relationship between the binary opposites intelligence and intellectual disability operates in both directions at once. Certain key moments in the historical emergence of learning disability as the template's chief occupant illustrate this.

One example – it seems obscure but do hold on, because it is a critical moment – comes from the early seventeenth century, when a concept of 'natural intellectual disability' lasting inevitably from birth to death first appeared. Its roots are political but also religious. Initially proposed by a dissident group of French Protestants, it formed part of their battle for converts against an oppressive Catholic state. They realized that their fellow Protestants' doctrine of predestination (God had determined prenatally who was elected for salvation and who were the hellbound reprobates) was hardly attractive. The state's Jesuit propagandists ridiculed it. How could an all-loving God be so nasty? Orthodox Protestants warned their dissident colleagues against making any concessions to the optimism of the Catholic Jesuits. Squeezed by these twin pressures, the radicals formed the hypothesis that certain individuals might exist who had an intellectual defect which Nature, not God, was the cause of, which lasted their whole lifetime and formed their identity. It was deterministic and unalterable, and could no longer be conceived as curable by providence, as previously. Unlike reprobates, however, these people were excused from God's judgment. From these small beginnings, this way of opposing ingroup and essential outgroup would soon overtake that between elect and reprobate.

Something similar happened in the English religious and educational culture too, and it was perhaps the most important foundation for modern intellectual ability and disability. Only once 'natural disability' had been thought up did the logical inference occur: a quasi-sacred *ability* might exist that was located entirely within 'natural man', a phrase that had formerly indicated a creature corrupted by original sin but now became something positive. This humanistic theory would help transform the minority Calvinist 'elect' into the Enlightenment ideal of humans as reasoners and, later, as the vast category of people of normal intelligence and above. The route to heaven now came from using one's own reason, alongside the odd bit of revelation. That is why it was a critical moment. More than philosophers, it was religious preachers and educators who, having eventually bowed before this principle on all sides of the religious spectrum, channelled it into the mainstream of cultural life in Western Europe and across the Atlantic.

Another historical example, a more or less direct offshoot of the first, came on the threshold of the modern psychological disciplines. At the start of the twentieth century a newly secular French state, replacing the inclusively minded Catholic church schools with a state education system, commissioned the psychologist Alfred Binet to help give it a rational structure. Rational structure meant categorization and segregation. Binet's absolute but unarticulated presupposition was that certain children have a deficiency in their very nature. As in the previous example, deficiency was *a priori*. He then pondered, deductively, a list of the things that might define it. And only via this process did he then start to identify a positive, intelligent counterpart. The latter, the normal population, went on to become the material for his first tests, in which he recalibrated the human part of the ladder of nature as the first modern intelligence scale. The tests' ultimate task, though, was to expose ('help') the deficient. The loop was thus completed and reinforced.

Binet's invention of mental age scores may have lent an air of precision and neutrality to the binary opposition, but his thought process clearly shows that he sculpted intelligence out of disability rather than the other way round. The researches of Lev Vygotsky, another landmark figure in the psychology of education (though he was opposed to the use of ability scales), followed a similar trajectory. His early researches, in a Soviet education system similarly caught up in secularization and modernization, were into what he called 'defectology' (the word has no value connotations in Russian). This fed directly into his later account of normal functions. Again, these then looped back finally, to help tighten his initially loose category of defectiveness.[7]

A third and more up-to-date example comes from current brain research and cognitive efficiency theory.[8] First, the absolute presupposition: that learning disability exists, as a psychological object or natural kind, together with the assumption that *slower* means deficient (speed and ease of learning are synonymous in cognitivist definitions of intelligence). Second comes the selection of certain people labelled already as having a learning disability, the hypothesis being that they will exhibit abnormally slow movements of neurons across synapses. Third, their slow movement is confirmed by observation. Fourth, they become the prior indicators by which the researcher is then able to establish a set of norms of correlation between the mental and the material (brain) components of the research. Fifth, this correlation is then used to pinpoint normal intelligence. Sixth, the norm, thus established as the stable reference-point, enables the researcher to go back and allocate more precise identifying characteristics to those who are deficient. Finally, the circularities are locked in by a standardized assessment. As an extra benefit, the scientific status of 'mind' within the mind–body duality has been reinforced.

Such circularities are again characteristic of a mindset dominated by inclusion phobia, in a state of abstract detachment that Gabel in his description of false consciousness calls autistic. The fact that the research subjects themselves are often people labelled with autism should not be thought of as simply ironic. Rather, it indicates that the autism category is a projection of the researchers' own state of mind.

Social construction and the social model

How we conceive of intellectual disability, then, plays an active role in how we conceive of intelligence. So in what sense are such differences a matter of social construction? The various versions of social construction theory – some stronger, some weaker – have in common a concern with identity and inequality. Dealing as they do with difference in a whole range of identities, when they do concern learning disability they borrow their language from those others – from race, gender, sexuality, etc. – as if people with learning difficulties were just another excluded group within the system, rather than one that actually defines the system as a whole by lying outside it and describing its boundaries.

The strong version of the theory sees the learning disability category as simply arbitrary – not only in historical terms but here and now. This occasionally rings true in real life. Sometimes a learning disability will be no more than the product of funding regimes (this has played a role for example in the recent rise of autism[9]). Whenever I visit a segregated school for children with severe learning difficulties, I can usually count on seeing a child who is completely normal by anyone's definition of the word, and who has drifted there perhaps owing to a variety of personal circumstances that fortuitously coincide with the host institution's need for numbers.

For example, I am shown round a summer playscheme at a school in a North London suburb. The headteacher tells me it is for 'complex needs and SLD', then, at a different point in the conversation, 'mainly autistic'. When the cut-off point for this or that type of special school was determined by IQ then at least you knew where you stood. The decline of IQ testing in school placement in favour of management fiat has provided an even greater licence to be creative. Evidence of this comes from 12-year-old Liam. He accompanies the headteacher and me on the mandatory school tour. He is the first to greet me, with 'It's nice to see you here' and then 'Not everybody is in because they said it's going to be the hottest day of the year today.' He has lots of sensible things to say about what we are looking at as we go through, though the headteacher blanks his fully social speech as if it's extraneous chatter. I have to doublecheck with her to confirm that he is on the school roll. Her explanation for his being there is that '80 per cent of the parents have got special needs themselves, they all live in the south-east of the borough' (the working-class area). When I probe for more detail, she says 'Poor parenting skills and things like that.'

I move on to another playscheme, a couple of miles away. There are no non-disabled children here, not even brothers and sisters. Some ten- and eleven-year-olds are in reins. Even within this segregated playground there is further segregation, a fenced-off area with a staff member permanently stationed at the combination lock. It has to be unlocked to let us in, and locked after us. It is not clear who is being protected, those inside or those outside. Two eleven-year-olds are pouring sand into buckets. 'We're making jam tarts,' says one. 'Can I have one?' I ask. 'They're pretend,' says his friend. Later I (stupidly) ask, 'Are you going to sell them to people?' 'They're pretend,' comes the exasperated reply again.

The strong version of the theory, then, asks 'Who is actually the idiot here?' However, it is usually the theory's weaker version that one encounters: something real lies beneath the learning disability label, but it can only be viewed through the prism of a particular social or cultural standpoint, since knowledge is 'not something people possess in their heads but rather something people do together'.[10] Indian railway stations, for example, are micro-cultures of the vulnerable and dispossessed, among whom people with microcephaly or Down's syndrome congregate. Living there as they please, they get casual support from fellow-citizens who would not accord it to the hundreds of other destitute wanderers.[11] A story widely reported at seminars on the developing countries tells of some earnest Western practitioners who, noting a lack of facilities for children with learning difficulties in Tanzania, set up a special school. Recruiting a teenager with Down's syndrome, they thought they had overcome his reluctant father, only for the boy to fail to show. Upon enquiry, the father's response was: 'If he's at school, who's going to help me run the shop?'

Who gets locked in a cage and who gets to run the shop has always depended on shared but shifting cultural meanings around status, as well as on the concrete social context and on the kind of life chances that everyone else is subject to, in any era. The weaker type of constructionism thus often evokes respect for other cultures, radicalism, optimism, or simply the human touch; nevertheless it usually leaves intact the presupposition that learning disability is an essential, cross-historical kind. Without a historical perspective to tell us that learning disability is a transient product of inclusion phobia, identifying intellectual difference as social construction may just be a way to have your cake and eat it. Citings of social theory have spread across the academic sector as routine signs of belonging, but those casual obeisances to Foucault, Derrida or Deleuze often deliver less than they promise. 'I'm a social constructionist,' comes the opening sentence from a clinical psychologist's paper in which she goes on to mourn the closure of the long-stay institutions. 'I'm with Deleuze and the rhizomes,' says the professor of nursing, in the middle of a stereotypically medical-model lecture on the ethics of pre-natal testing. 'I'm a *bricoleur*,' says a professor of education as he hedges his bets about the desegregation of schools.

This constructionist capacity for doublethink is deeply rooted. One example is Vygotsky again, or at least his followers. Human reasoning, they say, develops in the area between cultural contingency and the individual's primary biological nature, which they call the 'zone of proximal development.' This lies between what children can do with the guidance of others and what they can do on their own. The zone exists in learning disabled children too; it means they are educable, and might even have a possible route into the mainstream of life, if not into the intelligent ingroup as such.[12] Nevertheless, Vygotsky maintains that what they can do on their own is inextricable from the 'primary disorder' of their 'central nervous system' that causes their 'exclusion', and is skewed or impeded by this. Although he criticizes the principle of a fixed quantum of intelligence because it measures only an individual's performance and not their potential ability, he presupposes that the zone of proximal development, with or without added value from social and cultural contingencies, can apply in full only to normal children, i.e. those defined as having normal intelligence by the circular process described earlier. Vygotsky's premise is ultimately the same as that of the medical model; it locates the disorder and its fundamental description within the excluded person rather than, as the long historical perspective teaches us, in the excluder.

A second example is the medical model's official mouthpieces which, having for a long time rigorously ignored social explanations, have recently begun to make concessions to all those noisy constructionists. Both the World Health Organisation and the American Association on Intellectual and Developmental Disabilities now incorporate social risk factors, such as available levels of support, within their very definitions of intellectual disability.[13] In addition, the WHO has mainstreamed disability in general by situating it holistically alongside disease, mortality and poverty, in response to the political demands of physically disabled people. Nevertheless, with learning disability specifically, the concession to social constructionism is simply another episode in medical science's ongoing Up the Mountain story (good science drives out bad), whose lifeblood depends on keeping intact the underlying category. Socially defined elements of learning disability turn out to be a positive and useful tool after all: an injection of new blood into a jaded medical model.

The social model and the disability movement

A further example of the ambivalences in social construction is the very nature of the disability movement itself, dominated as it has been by activists with physical and sensory disabilities. Some propose to mainstream disability not via inclusion within existing social structures but by using the disabled identity to expand or renovate the mainstream. They reject the 'weakened strain of inclusionism' that suggests the excluded person can be included in a society that would otherwise remain as it is.[14] Disability is the metaphor for a conceptual disruption that would help reveal the infinity of human difference and thus demarginalize disability itself: a constructionist argument if ever there was one.[15] Disability in general is said to be not 'just another other' but itself a transformative category of analysis.[16] Yet neither physical nor sensory disability are fully implicated in the present phase of inclusion phobia, whose *extreme* outgroup exists above all in relation to intelligence because that is the core form of self-representation in modern species definition. At the same time, theoreticians and activists in the field tend to ignore or marginalize learning disability. This may be a good thing. It enables us to clarify the situation by separating the two. Seen from the long historical perspective of inclusion phobia, is learning disability an impairment at all?

Disability studies, as a discipline, routinely criticizes the modern era's tendency to think of the human being as a creature split into mind and body.[17] However, in other ways it falls for the very fallacy it criticizes. If (a) the disability movement's aim is to validate the impaired body and (b) disability is an umbrella term that covers both the physical and the mental, then the latter, if present in the argument at all, is only there as an afterthought. But perhaps it didn't fit in the first place. Of course learning disability sometimes has *some* connection to the materialities of physical impairment, inasmuch as the brain may be different.[18] Nevertheless, this sidesteps the issue. In the physically disabled person, the body as such is impaired. In the learning disabled person, an additional explanatory link is needed, between the (impaired) material substance of the brain and the (impaired?) immaterial intellect. The idea of brain-related learning disability recreates the problem (how human beings get to act at all) that mind–body dualism was meant to solve. There may be other ways entirely of looking at the problem. Pre-modern theories were not dualistic: the word stupid, for example, could refer indiscriminately and simultaneously to thought processes, to the material brain, and to the muscles it communicated with.

We should rather view the subordinate position of learning disability within the 'social model' of the disability movement and disability studies as being another effect of inclusion phobia. It is precisely by being capable of whatever it is the person with learning difficulties is *in*capable of that a black person's entry-ticket to the ingroup, or a woman's – both groups once deemed intellectually deficient by medical science – is valid, and the same is true for the physically disabled person. It is not so much that learning disability is a poor relation of physical within the disability category (though in terms of disability politics it is), rather that it is not a relation at all. The one does not differ from the other as a banana differs from an orange, but as a banana differs from a bandana. The phrases seem to be akin because of that word disability which they share, but as far as any intrinsic properties are concerned, the relationship is accidental.

The relationship takes various forms. Physical and learning disability sometimes occur in the same person – though cerebral palsy without learning disability still stands on an entirely different level of social status from cerebral palsy with it. If I had the average orienteering skills of someone with *either* motor-neurone disease *or* Down's syndrome, I wouldn't expect a job in air traffic control (though there have been and may in future be societies that do not have air traffic). And finally, both outgroups are subject to discrimination.

It is in this last respect that the divergence between the physical and the intellectual, for the practical purposes of the disability movement, starts to become clear. The excluded person with a physical disability does have a potential riposte to the question 'Does he take sugar?' which is, 'Why are you asking my friend instead of me? I'm not *stupid*.' Moreover, no one is going to lock up Mike Oliver, Emeritus Professor of Disability Studies at the University of Greenwich, just because he is not fully mobile without his wheelchair. But it can happen at any time, and without the right of appeal that even a mentally ill person has, to someone deemed to have a learning disability. It is characteristic of an extreme outgroup that there is no further outgroup along the chain to which the bucket can be passed.

The weak social constructionist theory of impairment roughly says that physical disability is a natural kind, upon which the social construction of disability is overlayered; there is a distinction between impairment (physical) and disability (socially imposed). More sophisticated analyses see impairment itself as incorporating social components.[19] The radically historical character of learning disability shows that it is not a natural kind, as we are about to see. Social construction in its weak sense says that interpretations of learning disability differ and no single one of them constitutes an absolute truth: historical interpretations and reinterpretations of it, therefore, are relative, while the thing itself, the impairment, retains a more or less hidden reality. Social construction in the strong sense means relativizing actual abilities: the word impairment therefore loses its underlying reality even within the present. However, as certain abilities are necessary to the particular society one lives in, to relativize them in this way would be to leave people without them floundering. In the latter sense learning disability is certainly no 'mere' social construction. But it *is* specifically modern, even if its sketchiest origins go back many centuries.

The need for a workable historical method

If theories of social construction cannot entirely account for learning disability, would 'historical construction' be a better description? This phrase is normally used in a similar way: it says that history is 'a fable agreed upon' rather than a 'reporting [of] the past'.[20] For the purposes of this book, however, I *am* using it in this latter sense; I am reporting on past behaviours as an anthropologist would report on contemporary customs, and treating difference, in the case of extreme outgroups, as an abstract template whose concrete details are filled in not by the history of learning disability but by the history of inclusion phobia. There was and is already a general template there to be filled, and to discover how this works is the job of the historian as much as anybody else, inasmuch as (to quote Roger Smith) 'without historical knowledge of the beliefs held about the nature of being human we are ignorant of what it is to be human'.[21]

In the case of the present era, the intelligence society's failure to acknowledge its own history is part of an irrationality that would be exposed if it turned out that learning disability was not a fixed item in nature but merely a temporary historical occupant of the template. Unravelling the irrationality demands that we find a workable historical method. And there is in fact one readily available in the history of medicine. When we examine texts from the past, we have to remember that while labels are one thing, definitions and lists of characteristics are another. They have to be separated from each other. Avoiding retrospective diagnosis is an elementary precaution. If you look up tonsilitis in the index of a Renaissance medical compendium, how do you know that it indicates an inflammation of the throat? Why not the big toe? This may seem like quibbling. Take another term, then. Phrenitis, inflammation of the brain, comes from an ancient Greek word for the diaphragm (*phren*), and its symptoms have wandered all over the body in between times. Historians of bodily disease probe the descriptive characteristics that surround any such term in the main text, and do not take for granted that it means now what it meant then. Only with labels apparently equivalent to learning disability do historians feel confident enough to skip this rudimentary precaution and go hunting for cross-historical idiots as if the symptomatic content of their difference were a permanent and indisputable fact.

Using such a method immediately reveals certain premises on which a framework for the future might be built too. On the one hand you would not have needed a WAIS score of 40 or above to have a job helping with the ancient

Sumerian harvest, or to negotiate your way like everyone else around the village or small town where you lived. On the other hand learning disability is, for the time being, something real: it belongs to the living and working arrangements, technologies and general social organization of our particular era. Hence a learning disabled person's explanation of how to get to the moon is not as reliable as a rocket scientist's.

Comparing across centuries, however, abilities *can* turn out to be relative. If that ancient Sumerian did not need the equivalent of a normal IQ to work in the fields, in modern societies you do sometimes need a university degree to work in a call centre. Learning disability is not an impairment in the longer time-frame, in the way that a missing limb might always have been. 'If we were cavemen, we'd be fine,' as one researcher was told.[22] I am cheating slightly, as this particular student was dyslexic and did not have learning difficulties in the sense covered by this book; he was talking about the irrelevance, in an era of computer technologies for learning and personal wikis for communication, of the speculative psycho-medical cures for which cognitive genetics programmes are funded.[23] Nevertheless, if what he said can apply to a specific problem like dyslexia, which is a historical outcome only of mass literacy, it can apply to learning disability in general, a concept that is equally a product of stretched social relations, of empire and complex urbanization. The irrelevance of cure applies in a broadly similar way to both past and future circumstances, as long as any future technology is also rooted in ordinary human decencies such as 'active listening' and 'establishing rapport'.[24]

The long time-frame can be represented visually as a bell curve. If the *x* axis represents the passage of centuries from the past into the future, and the *y* axis the socially constructed prevalence of learning disability, the latter peaks at the present historical moment and tends at either end to zero. Inclusion phobia, by contrast, being a constant – near-universal and permanent – can be represented as a horizontal line. Or so it seems. It is not impossible to imagine a future in which the development of technology means that learning disability is no longer with us, but that would not be as a result of its being *cured*, as a natural kind; it would have something to do with changes to the target on which inclusion phobia has set its sights. Eliminating the phobia itself is another matter, and is a political and ethical question that goes beyond the scope of this present book. Nevertheless, it would be the more appropriate and achievable goal for anyone wanting to change the world for people with learning difficulties and themselves.

Comparative psychology and the ladder of nature

In short, an existing and quite routine historical method reveals that learning disability has a point of onset within the human cultural past, albeit one spread over centuries. In the short term it shifts within certain conceptual boundaries that continue to be recognizable for a while, but in the medium to long term it transcends them. As in the previous chapter, we can track that history at the higher, philosophical level first, that of the ladder of nature. We saw where and how human intelligence is located on this ladder. The place of learning disability on it, as a fundamental expression of inclusion phobia, is likewise premised on a fear of animality.

Biologists have attempted to dismantle the notion of a hierarchical ladder, beginning with the nineteenth century's final detachment of biological science from religion. It featured the arrival of comparative psychology, a subdiscipline whose starting assumption was that human and animal intelligence share some common denominator. As biologist Stuart Firestein writes, the idea of a ladder of nature is a downgrading of animals.[25] In this respect, he says, science still carries an unfortunate historical baggage of religion and morals. Animals 'have to perform at nearly superhuman levels to be even considered as having something we might call "mind", whatever that is.' Even more perceptively, he writes 'what we call mind tends to be circularly defined as something that humans have'. The negative starting assumption, that animals don't think, puts all the onus on them to prove that they do.

However, the ladder proves not so easy to kick away. This concession to animal intelligence comes at the expense of something or someone else. Firestein, distancing himself from the 'we' in what follows, argues that

> the threshold for showing cognitive abilities in animals is much higher than it is for humans, even obviously damaged humans with severe mental dysfunction. No matter how retarded a child may be, we still believe he or she has essential human qualities, including a cognitive life that is soul-like.

His scepticism about the ladder of nature gets momentarily suspended as 'retarded' humans lie, it might be suggested, *below* animals. Mind ('whatever that is') is a floppy concept, he says – but when he needs to identify an outgroup *lacking* it, suddenly there it is in all its glory. Firestein's thought process is an illustration of Gabel's theory about the structural identity between schizophrenia and ideology. His scepticism about the ladder of nature gets momentarily suspended as 'retarded' humans are posited *below* animals. This was already a stock procedure from the start of modern concepts of learning disability. Locke, for example, insisted that we have to be sceptical about whether the place of the human species on the ladder can be defined by the possession of 'reason' as his predecessors had defined it, but only so that he could exclude the congenitally deficient who have 'less [reason] than a cockle or an oyster' from the new definition of reason that he wanted to propose instead.[26]

Before that, in the era of early empire, outgroups in general were defined loosely. Social complexity was managed by the incorporation of functional (albeit still hierarchical) parts within an integrated social whole; this included even obvious outgroups such as slaves. Fools, meanwhile, were not an obvious group at all. Among the Romans, the word most often used (*morio*) could describe anyone aspiring to a respect or status that others were unwilling to accord them. Its defining characteristics might be a wonky nose, or inept table manners. It was also the job title of your household jester, whether or not he had any cognitive deficiencies in the modern sense; or it could be you, the master, if for example you enjoyed watching him have sex with your wife.[27] In religion St Augustine, under that same Latin label, entirely reinvents them each time for the sake of whatever theological context he is citing them in; they have the common function of innocently offsetting the vices of fallen humanity, but the characteristics he gets them to exhibit are always quite different. In short, we are looking at a very broad concept indeed, and mostly an unrecognizable one. We do come across stray references to cognitive criteria of a sort at this time. If you were blind, you might be unable to see geometrical forms; this would demote you intellectually because you would be incapable of grasping the founding intellectual principle that the mind was the 'form' of the body's 'matter'. And if you were deaf, unable to hear words that stand for particular things, you would be unable to group them together into abstract categories. But these were just secondary aspects of sensory impairment as such.

It was in the late medieval era that the ladder of nature took hold. Doctrine still held that only the outermost and faintest of the nine angelic circles of the Intellect had any connection to the human realm. The idea that human beings lie midway between the animal and the divine and aspire to the latter is so deeply embedded in us that usually we are unaware of its presence. And because the animals are below us on the ladder (unlike in some cultures where animals can be equal partners), we suffer vertigo: there but for the grace of God go I. And in this hierarchical scale that runs downward from our own would-be divinity to the sheer animal nature beneath, a rung seems to be missing. In aspiring to that realm above, we are also making a panicky escape from that dangerous slot below. From the middle ages onwards, this delusional anxiety has placed there a variety of types, whose inferiority is conceived in three ways: as difference by degree within the same species, as an interstitial difference between two species (usually between humans and monkeys), or as an anomaly. It was from the last of these that the idea of abnormality associated with modern learning disability arose; unlike the first two types of difference, anomaly suggested something *outside* nature altogether and therefore demonic or evil.

In short, there was an *a priori* slot for creatures who are only quasi-human and therefore animal-like. It therefore had to be filled by something. As Moore points out, entire categories such as 'heretic' or 'leper' were largely invented. They were products of the elite imagination, projections of its fear of dirt that led to their being bracketed with animals literally, rather than metaphorically like the multitudes lacking a landed estate or professional qualifications. Reason had been an aspect of divinity which human beings could aim at despite being bogged down in their animal existence; but once the validity of a purely natural and specifically human reason began to be acceptable, the inference could be drawn that there might be individual exceptions to the rule, and that a proper system for categorizing them might be needed as backup.

The ladder of nature: modern rearrangements

The late seventeenth century, as we saw, was a watershed in this respect. It had been preceded by certain necessary historical developments. On top of the firming up of administrative categories in the late middle ages, the Reformation came to see God's relationship with man as being rather with individuals than with the species as a whole. Together, these developments exposed personal deficiencies whose acknowledged existence had not previously challenged the fixed definition of the species. Individuals in this disaggregated sense then had to be accounted for. In 1689 the Glorious Revolution secured legitimacy for Protestant occupancy of the English throne but also for the theoretical roots of modern democracy. In addition to writing one of the foundational texts of modern psychology, Locke also laid out the revolution's core political ideology.[28] In adding the principles of rational consent and individual autonomy to that of logical reasoning as the essence of human identity, this work refined and pathologized the definition of idiocy accordingly. Published within a few months of each other, Locke's two seminal works, one about the mind and the other about politics, were faces of the same coin. Between them, they established for the modern mindset what it is to be human. The dominant strand in political philosophy today, which sees the very basis of democracy, citizenship and human rights as our intellectual ability to consent, regards human beings as having been invented at the Battle of the Boyne.[29] In this excluding assumption, rational autonomy, underpinned by cognitive capacity, is man's 'original position' in the state of nature.

The assertion of an original state of any kind involves the denial of history typical of inclusion phobia. In fact 'the concept of being human itself has a history', and it is a much longer one than that.[30] The answer to 'What is a human being?' for the Greeks had been that it's obvious and generally accepted: it is a creature born of human parents and sharing a physical resemblance with other human beings. Medieval thinkers stuck to this, though as well as being generally accepted it was also what the Pope said it was. Locke thought that religious absolutism of this sort, like political absolutism, treated adult human beings as subservient idiots. His answer was, instead, that the human species is an aggregate of non-idiotic individuals whose resemblance to each other lies in their ability, each for themselves, to reason. He set out the detailed empirical processes that enable us to think logically and to make abstractions from sense data. In his definition of human reason, the possession of innate 'common ideas' was replaced by the possession of innate operations of the mind. Breaking with his medieval predecessors, he believed that all of us possess these operations, irrespective of gender, class or race (albeit with some ambiguity in the latter two instances). Everyone is to be trusted and politically tolerated to work out their own intellectual pathway towards perfection via the detailed workings of certain mental processes they all have in common.

From here comes the idea of a few exceptional individuals who test and contradict that principle. Their very existence secures the external boundary of the ingroup, of that 'everyone' which now thinks it is the species. The picture works by pointing us to the threat of a few fake look-alikes who lie outside the ingroup, that is to say, below it on the ladder of nature. The anxiety is not (as it is with mental illness) about who is rational and who not, but about their species membership. Locke promoted a new definition of what it is to be human precisely in order to make people more aspirational. His aim was religious, and only secondarily democratic: every individual should prepare, intellectually and morally, for the second coming. Medieval talk about the beastlike nature of idiots, when the word had meant the lower classes in general, had been largely figurative; Locke's turn towards describing universal operations of the mind, at the same time as reducing the numbers of the bestial, injected a new seriousness into the categorization of the outgroup and the threat it posed to those preparations. He suggested as a future project dividing it up into sub-categories according to their different 'ways of faltering' – a suggestion not taken up till two centuries later.

Another way in which Locke pointed forward to the modern disciplines lay in his suggestion that deficiencies in intelligence, rather than (as previously) physical deformity, might be grounds for infanticide. Following in Locke's foot-steps, Peter Singer made a much publicized recommendation (later modified) for the euthanasia of live infants with Down's syndrome on the grounds of their intelligence. Some animals might be more intelligent.[31] As I write, New York State judges are deciding whether Tommy the Chimp has the rights and status of a person. Promoting chimpanzees to personhood is an entirely logical out-come of 1689, and marks an especially aggressive phase of inclusion phobia's schizoid thought processes. Animality after all is what the ingroup is trying to escape, yet here it is pulling animals on board. In a reversal of their relative positions on the ladder of nature before the modern era, Tommy the Chimp is almost human, Tommy the man with Down's syndrome almost not. What started off as metaphor – certain humans are like animals – not only becomes literal but is exacerbated so that some actual animals are above those humans on the ladder. They are raised to personhood in the same breath as some humans are denied it and eliminated.

This self-contradiction demonstrates the element of *persecution*, as Girard notes, in inclusion phobia. Contamination disgust thus lies at the root not only of the modern categorization of learning disability but also of today's eugenics. When Locke expressed disgust at the sight of 'your driveling, unintelligent, intractable changeling', it was more than one man's OCD quirk.[32] It chimed with a whole new social mentality that would eventually come up with eugenics and the segregated institutions. Sharper categorizations of difference helped reconceptualize the norm, and to see intelligence now as the property of a broad aggregate of the population including most members of a previously beast-like multitude. It was Locke's small minority of excluded individuals that enabled him to assume a starting equality in the basic reasoning of the rest, a huge ingroup whose intellectual differentiations within the band of normal now operate independently of differentiations in social status (in theory, if not in practice). Modern meritocracy and its glittering promises were achieved through the conceptualization of a remainder to whom the disability label is now attached, and at their expense.

Outgroups before modern psychology

We saw in the previous chapter how the ladder of nature was also embedded in everyday considerations of status and the making of bids for esteem. As late as 1600, honour and grace were still *the* desirable personal qualities, but during a seventeenth-century lifetime, a specifically human reason, viewed in an entirely positive light, would begin to feature in this same class of subjective, inborn qualities. And if it was from interaction among all three that modern ideas of intelligence sprang, so too did learning disability. While today we define it by those cognitive characteristics such as inability to process information, think abstractly or reason logically, an equivalent-sounding label from before 1600 – 'natural fool,' for example – displayed a totally different set. Natural fools could be marked by a penchant for dressing up, proneness to catarrh, licentious behaviour, or denying the existence of God. What are we to make of such a strange, disparate list? The first item refers to the occupational role of court and household jesters who may well have been no stupider than their masters; the second to ancient medical theory, in which mental states were secondary organic facets of physical disease; the last two to moral panics about atheism. The behaviours describing the natural fool were dishonourable and graceless: they transgressed social and religious norms that were very much of their time, not ours.

It is not the odd natural fool with strange behaviour but the great mass of the vulgar and the damned who are the precursors of the modern disabled person. In social and religious terms, the honourable and the elect defined their status by singling it out from the contaminating, brutish herd who worked with their hands, dealt with money or had no profession, or who were reprobates determined by God for hell before they were born. References to information-processing, abstraction and mental logic do, as we have seen, appear in medieval theories of the mind. If the men servicing those institutions could boast the management skills such as these that would eventually define modern intelligence, who was it who lacked them?

The medieval clerical caste disdained the illiterate. Moore cites mental speed and familiarity with new administrative techniques involving the law (and lucre, though being filthy it was unmentionable in such contexts) as the stimulus for the rise of reason. However, this still seems to leave open the idea that an objective realm of human intellect already existed in nature, waiting for upcoming generations to draw on, when in fact it was no more than a professional cachet: an internalization of those techniques as psychological objects. Taking this into account would add sharpness to Moore's picture of a 'the hostility of the *clericus* towards the *illiteratus, idiota, rusticus*'. The Latin words have started to mean what you think they do; they are forming a language in which inclusion phobia was beginning to crystallize around a new core:

> The fear which was expressed in the language of contamination, directed against the poor in general and in particular against heretics, lepers, Jews, prostitutes, vagrants and others assimilated to them by the rhetoric of persecution, was the fear which the *literati* harboured of the *rustici*. No doubt it assisted many of them to identify themselves more securely with the privilege to which their skills had brought them access, by entrenching and justifying the exclusion of those who lacked them.[33]

Over the centuries, those social and external exclusions became built into the foundations of Western thought, as an aspect of some subjective, internal nature: the category of a quasi-human type whose *essence* was to *lack* reason.

Sometimes the skills were lacking in their superiors too. Clerks would scold their noble employers for their illiteracy, or else use their skills to rob them blind. Largely, though, the fact that the word idiot denoted illiterates or lay people in general tells us that abilities which modern cognitive science sees as characteristically human were perceived as absent by definition in the masses. If a gentleman's honourable station just *was* a superiority denoting indiscriminately both intellectual ability and social power (a landed estate), so too, to lack one kind of ability was to lack the other: they were overlapping concepts. We can see from sixteenth-century paintings that if there were exceptional cases, these were related to social class in terms of people's physiognomy. In the Vienna Kunstmuseum is a famous portrait of a woman carrying the name Elizabeth the Stupid. She is dressed appropriately to her noble status. Her face is odd, but only in the context of the idealized portraits alongside it; unless we are determined to stick with retrospective diagnosis, it is not medicalized. What she *does* look like is a Brueghel peasant. And this means, not that Brueghel painted peasants as if they were fools, but that someone labelled stupid in an aristocratic setting would have been perceived as peasant-like. Exceptions aside, intellectual ability was assumed *within* the material ability of the upper social ranks. Thus, according to a widely read behavioural manual of the time, the corresponding mark of disability was the absence of social 'aids and supports ... measured by the credit, want, company, conceit, or instability of the person' – in short, the social model, well ahead of its current but similar manifestation as 'the expression of limitations in individual functioning within a social context'.[34]

We can track some of this in the social history of specific social groups or even actual individuals. Girard's 'crisis of differentiation' is relevant again here. The values of the clerical caste attracted the growing number of competitive town-dwellers from outside the feudal landholding system, who formed an emergent urban bourgeoisie. This fluidity led to a point in the mid-seventeenth century when the difference between ingroup and outgroup was in that acute, mobile stage which inclusion phobia sometimes exhibits. The Levellers, early advocates of universal (male) suffrage, explicitly excluded both servants and country gentry from this, since both groups were uncivil and thus idiotic. Their elite opponents, confronted with bottlenecks in social mobility for their younger sons, started to abandon old prejudices and put them to apprenticeship or business. There could now be city gents (i.e. traders) as well as landed ones.

Ongoing crises of differentiation in social status were at first complemented but then superseded by those of religious status. In the early seventeenth century many people had been overwhelmed with anxiety about their state of grace. Death of the soul (still roughly synonymous with 'mind') was a greater horror than the death of the body. Since God had already decided before you were even conceived whether you were bound for heaven or on a one-way ticket to hell, people were desperate to know which box they fell into. This Calvinist law of predestination was akin to today's genetic determinism: nothing you did could alter your fate. Reprobates were marked by their inability to reason, but this meant an inability to rationally examine their consciences for the signs of grace; in everyday affairs, they were assumed to function normally. So on the one hand their lack of intelligence again bore little resemblance to how we define learning disabled people today, while on the other hand they were especially dangerous because you could not tell they belonged to the extreme outgroup just by looking at them. Thus the anxiety around them anticipates early twentieth-century 'morons', or Singer's reluctance to let human-ness be just a matter of physical appearance.

There could, however, be proxy signs of reprobation which led to physical segregation. In the middle ages, the lay population were largely allocated to the nave; Aquinas stipulated that illiterate laypeople (*idiotae*) could not receive holy communion. Even in the mid-seventeenth century, sleeping or yawning during sermons could get you barred. So too could an inability to understand the catechism. A good Protestant's understanding of the eucharist was metaphorical and therefore reasoned or 'intellectual', contrasting it with the simplistic and idolatrous nature of transubstantiation. Strictly speaking, then, earthly administrators could endanger your salvation by barring you from the rite, though till now it had been assumed that you could be readmitted by amending your behaviour or, in the case of the mentally ill, by having lucid intervals. It was out of debate over such matters that some ecclesiastical authorities came to construct 'idiots' of a more modern-looking kind. The extreme outgroup template demanded the existence of a group of people whom one would know instinctively to exclude without even submitting them to the tests applied to everyone else. Their incurable deficiency – alongside but not overlapping with that of reprobates – was of a determinate and birth-to-death nature.

From categories to cages

Even in the first half of the nineteenth century, the idea of reprobation remained alive and well alongside that of a natural social hierarchy. Jane Eyre, for example, sees her schoolmistress' job as being to rescue a handful of her young peasant charges from the swamps of both vulgarity *and* damnation. Only once the mid-century knowledge elite had turned towards a biology that could do without religious props did modern idiots arrive, as properly scientific items, and with them the first large segregated institutions. Modern psychiatry had started to emerge, taking off from an old polarity between wildness and civilization. With the Enlightenment, older stories had begun to resurface of children reared by bears or wolves coming out from the forest, and of attempts to educate them. Their culmination was Victor, the Wild Boy of Aveyron,[35] a famous case that inspired some of the first medical and psychiatric pioneers to emerge from the French revolution, with its defence (by guillotine if necessary) of the purity of reason. The revolutionary ideology of Jacobinism was itself in part a legacy of Catholic versions of the election/reprobation doctrine. Zealous divisiveness was therefore in these psychiatrists' blood. The subtitle of the most reliable book about Victor calls him 'the last wild child and the first mentally deficient one' (*premier enfant fou*, the French descriptor having a wider application than the English one).[36] Victor, having achieved worldwide fame, remains a focal point for retrospective diagnoses of learning disability or latterly autism.

Medical science, having expressed little interest in idiots (however defined) before 1800 or so, now competed with the legal profession to take over practical arrangements. Britain's first long-stay hospital, the Royal Earlswood Asylum for Idiots, was the brainchild of Dr John Connelly, who drove forward new schematic medical definitions of idiocy and imbecility that accompanied his enthusiasm for segregated provision. Charles Dickens visited the newly built asylums.[37] His ideal of a mass citizenry aspiring towards respectability was unable to do without an outgroup, leading him to view the new institutions through an idealistic lens of philanthropic approval, as aids to social progress. It is a continuing peculiarity of inclusion phobia that benevolence and obsessive compulsion about ingroup cleanliness are two sides of the same coin. The seeds of this can be seen at least as far back as the Renaissance writer Juan Luis Vives, claimed by both welfarism and psychiatry as an early pioneer. Recommending the transference of relief from individual almsgivers to public authorities, he also insisted on new kinds of treatment for the 'furious' and the 'stupid'. On the one hand they should not be mocked, on the other they should not be permitted in public spaces such as church; he used as his analogy here the human body, which in ejecting its waste matter into sewers thereby helps to prevent corruption of the mind.

Intertwined cultural and scientific theories of evolution, progress and development of the mid-nineteenth century arrived, in part, *thanks to* these newly coined cross-historical idiots. A recasting of outgroups has helped recast the ingroup as scientific reasoners. In fact the majority of people we would now identify as learning disabled were not in institutions (and never have been), while very many of those who were there would not be identified as learning disabled today. It is no surprise, then, that relevant forms of advocacy, challenging both concept and practice, are as old as the institutions themselves. Even before Royal Earlswood, and covering 'idiots' too, there was an Alleged

Lunatics' Friend Society (note the constructionist angle in that adjective) which tried to prevent unwarranted confinements in the small asylums and work-houses of the time.[38] Some historians have noted a progress from benevolence to neglect in the regimes of segregated institutions, while others prefer to see them (especially schools) as getting better and better. In fact there has been no unidirectional shift either way, rather an ongoing tension between community and confinement.

Outside the walls of the asylum, ordinary life has for some people been not even an aspiration, just a fact of life, as the above examples from India and Tanzania, as well as Western examples from before the modern era, testify.[39] As well as advocacy, person-centred planning minus the name has probably been a constant too. Yet historians have tended to focus on the history of institutional segregation, and while this has turned up invaluable sources it draws attention away from the conceptual history.[40] The unwitting consequence of this focus is to reinforce the category and thus make it more likely that people today will remain ensnared in conceptual and thus institutional segregation than they otherwise might have been. The phrase 'out of sight, out of mind' takes on a dynamic significance. Critical historians are as guilty of this as anyone else. While there is a positivist world view that sees people with learning difficulties as a hindrance to its goals, there is also an equally negative but anti-positivist one which says there is nothing you can do to counter this.

Moore, for example, sees the tightened categories around medieval anti-semitism and leprosy as the catalytic precursor of a European history heading for the punitive incarcerations typical of modern power. Learning disability, as a historically specific manifestation of inclusion phobia, is absent from his picture. Regardless of the interpenetration between the conceptual and institutional aspects of difference, it is important to make the effort of separating the conceptual ones out first. The answer as to their invisibility lies in the rational quadrangles of the academy itself. The increasing demonization of innate lack of intelligence is a structural component of the very human science disciplines that might also help us to identify it. The mentally ill, however feeble their social supports, have partly succeeded in putting relativism on the agenda; at least they have got the academy and even psychiatry itself to agree that sanity can only be defined as lack of insanity. Try doing that with intelligence. It is intellectual difference specifically, however construed, that has come to form the core outgroup whose absences, by their very existence, define and etch in the entire present age of intelligent meritocracy. Moreover, the sources of that phobia are not popular prejudice or folklore but the elite cultures of the medieval and early modern periods, whose direct legacy the modern human sciences are.

The modern discipline could not have formalized its specific ingroup, the intelligent, without specifying (sometimes first of all) an outgroup of the entirely non-intelligent. Without reprobates to admonish, you could not be elect; without the vulgar to be admired by, you could not be honourable; and so, without the intellectually disabled to pathologize and segregate, you cannot be intelligent.

Even those who will agree that intelligence is a purely relative notion do not apply this to learning disability, especially when pronounced to be severe. If intelligence is not the same thing existing throughout history, how can learning disability be? How can 'people with learning difficulties' be a real category? And if it is not, what are we supposed to do with that knowledge, in practical terms?

Whether a bid for status comes through grace, honour or intelligence, it has as its core ideal to be well born and well bred (that was the etymological root of the word eugenics, and remains its core meaning). Successful bidders project a pathological phobia of contamination on to certain of their fellow human beings, whom they then exclude, segregate or eliminate. Codifying and updating status differentials into the relevant 'natural' and supposedly value-free format of the day is a way of building protective barriers against a swamp of social dirt and mortality. People with learning difficulties are of course entirely absent from all debate about meritocracy and social mobility. Again, their absence is not *mere* absence or overlooking, it is the keystone in the whole meritocratic edifice and its motives.

Of course some types of mental performance can be empirically verified, and will thus always yield the same results. An ancient Babylonian, a modern practitioner, even perhaps a Martian, would score them the same. But verification is one kind of thought-process: it is a *judgment* of something that lies outside ourselves. Choosing a category, labelling it intelligence or intellectual disability and deciding which discrete types of performance to include under that heading, is a another kind of thought-process entirely: it is a *sorting of terms*, which originates in our own heads and varies according to who is controlling the discussion or what the consensus is. Confuse a judgment with a sorting of terms, and you allow the hard, cross-historical reality of the first to underwrite the consensual, temporary reality of the second. And whatever applies to intelligence in this sense applies to learning disability no less. Later chapters will reveal the hard bargaining about what (and what not) to include that has gone into the sorting and fixing of a category such as autism. This too is a temporary cultural creation, very much of its time, like the more general learning disability paradigm; both override the uniqueness of the individual and lead down the path to social segregation. A conceptual box becomes a physical one, with a lid. It stays shut and hides abuse.

Learning disability in the concrete historical totality

Having looked at some of the detail, we finally get to see where learning disability sits in the history of inclusion phobia as a 'concrete totality', to use Gabel's phrase. For a historically specific understanding of inclusion phobia, we have to try and avoid being simplistic about its overall structures. For example, the idea of intellectual disability as a paradigmatic difference above all others works for the modern era not just because intelligence and rational autonomy are currently central to the fixing of social status in nature, but also because of modernity's espousal of a single progressive pathway *per se*. Its place belongs specifically in the idea of a universal history of humankind, an idea that dates back no further than Kant or at the earliest Bacon. The idea of a *single* paradigmatic case would not work for preceding eras, because they lacked the modern notion of a unity of earthly purpose and utilitarian means. And that, among other things, is why it is important to know about them. It helps us to perceive the schizoid denial of history in the dominant ideology of intelligence.

To view the historical shifts in their concrete totality, it is necessary to juggle the long term, the medium term and the short term, and to focus on (a) the *specificities* of (b) *conceptual* history while (c) identifying *evolving* patterns rather than mere 'snapshots', as Patrick McDonagh warns, of a particular era.[41] Thus we avoid the twin perils of grand but unspecific theory on the one hand and positivism with retrospective diagnosis on the other. We can grasp intellectual difference only once we observe *all* extreme or core outgroups in their proper historical context and look at its place within or alongside them.

The outgroups of medieval Jews, lepers and heretics shared certain paradigmatic characteristics that made them all of the extreme type, but had others that made them distinct from each other. There was in fact no single, unitary outgroup. The roots of the Jewish identity may (or may not – the point is hotly disputed[42]) have been as much socially and historically contingent as biological; but be that as it may, anti-semitism was intrinsic to the medieval economy and politics in a way that it is not today. As for heresy, something broadly similar applies but different again in its detail; the chief form of heresy, Catharism, was largely the invention of the inquisitors.[43] In the long historical term, there could not have been the idea that Jews or Cathars were deficient unless there had already been an underlying and more general concept of extreme difference in the first place, a template which, say, reprobates or idiots would also fill at various points – mainly later, but sometimes coinciding with or overlapping the former groups.

Difference is not an abstraction that transcends historical particulars. Concepts of human difference in history must therefore be carefully nuanced. This applies particularly to the Nazi analogy as used by critics of bioethical approaches to learning disability like Singer's. The mad, phobic aberration of the Holocaust and twentieth-century anti-semitism, like its current manifestations, was the residue of a specific disorder that had ceased for centuries to be vital to the functioning of the economy or the society and its forms of self-representation and status. Rarely, moreover, is the Holocaust referred to as a euthanasia programme. That, however, is what we call the Nazi project for eliminating the disabled, suggesting that it was simply the questionable application of an otherwise justifiable urge. The murder of around 200,000 'feeble-minded' people from the late 1930s, with even less of a murmur raised outside Germany than inside, was not a *trial run* for the extermination of religious others as it is often presented. It was certainly the first version of a gassing technology that was later refined on a mass scale for the Jews; nevertheless, the inspiration behind it was not merely an equivalent component of the Holocaust alongside anti-semitism, and was certainly not an afterthought. It was the forethought.[44] To begin with, incurable mental deficiency was the *whole point* of eugenic ideology and practice. Only subsequently did the Nazis digress to eliminate racial and religious groups by more general criteria. In fact the very first eugenic moves targeted the physically unfit, but the aim here was sterilization rather than extermination. Death was first mooted for the feeble-minded, and that was because learning disability alone had come to fill the extreme outgroup template.

I have described above the *transitions* from one constellation of outgroups to another, and thus how learning disability came to fill the central slot, under various names, as the modern era's essential difference. 'Essential' in the sense that if outgroups at the outset of the early modern era – the uneducated working classes, women, and ethnic and religious minorities – have succeeded in removing their historical taint of a deficient starting intelligence (and of course it remains a big if), they leave behind that residuum, people with learning disabilities, and will even stake their whole claim to ingroup membership on being not like them. The elevation of the Holocaust to a meta-narrative of scapegoating and persecution in general has thus scotched inclusion phobia, not killed it. Learning disability remains the undrained sump from which other forms of dehumanization can always draw.

Notes

1 See for example E. Zigler and R. Hodapp (1986). *Understanding Mental Retardation.* Cambridge: Cambridge University Press.
2 See J. A. Plucker and A. Esping (eds) (2015). 'Human intelligence: historical influences, current controversies, teaching resources'. www.intelltheory.com. Retrieved 28 November 2014.
3 G. Canguilhem (1989). *The Normal and the Pathological.* New York: Zone.
4 Girard, *The Scapegoat*, p. 21.
5 See Chapter 5.
6 T. Booth and M. Ainscow (2002). *Index for Inclusion: Developing Learning and Participation in Schools.* Bristol: CSIE.
7 L. Zankov (1936), 'Foreword to Vygotsky's developmental diagnostics and educational clinic of difficult childhood', cited in K. Rodina (2006). *Vygotsky's Social Constructionist View on Disability: A Methodology for Inclusive Education.* UCLA San Diego Laboratory of Comparative Human Cognition. www.lchc.ucsd.edu/MCA/paper. Retrieved 2 December 2014.
8 See for example Columbia University Medical Centre, http://newsroom.cumc. columbia.edu/blog/2014/08/21/children-autism-extra-synapses-brain/ Retrieved 2 December 2014.
9 See Chapter 8.
10 K. Gergen (1985). 'The social constructionist movement in modern psychology', *American Psychologist* 40, 266–375.
11 M. Miles (2010). *The Chuas of Sha Daulah at Gujrat, Pakistan: Evidence, Historical Background and Development, with Bibliography, 1839–2009.* Stockholm: Independent Living Institute. P. Balasundaram (2005). *Sunny's Story.* Delhi: ISPCK.
12 L. Vygotsky (1978). *Mind in Society: The Development of Higher Psychological Processes.* Cambridge, MA: Harvard University Press.

13 R. Schalock et al. (2010). *Intellectual Disability: Definition, Classification and Systems of Support*. Washington, DC: AAIDD.

14 D. Mitchell with S. Snyder (2015). *The Biopolitics of Disability: Neoliberalism, Ablenationalism, and Peripheral Embodiment*. Ann Arbor: University of Michigan Press.

15 M. Shildrick (2009). *Dangerous Discourses of Disability, Subjectivity and Sexuality*. New York: Palgrave Macmillan.

16 C. Kudlick (2003). 'Disability history: why we need another other', *American Historical Review* 108(3), 763–793.

17 B. Hughes and K. Patterson (1997). 'The social model of disability and the disappearing body: towards a sociology of impairment', *Disability and Society* 12(3), 325–340; K. Patterson (1999) 'Disability studies and phenomenology: the carnal policies of everyday life', *Disability and Society* 14(5), 597.

18 T. Shakespeare (2006). *Disability Rights and Wrongs*. Abindgdon: Routledge. S. Vehmas and P. Mäkelä (2008) 'The ontology of disability and impairment: a discussion of the natural and social features,' in K. Kristiansen et al., *Arguing about Disability: Philosophical Perspectives*, 42–56. Abingdon: Routledge.

19 D. Goodley (2001). '"Learning difficulties", the social model of disability and impairment: challenging epistemologies', *Disability and Society* 16(2), 207–231.

20 J. Meiland (1965). *Scepticism and Historical Knowledge*. New York: Random House, p. vi.

21 R. Smith (2007). *Being Human: Historical Knowledge and the Creation of Human Nature*. New York: Columbia University Press.

22 O. Barden (2012), 'Facebook as a catalyst for critical literacy learning by dyslexic sixth-form students', *Literacy* 46(3), 123–132.

23 See for example P. Wolff et al. (1996). 'Family patterns of developmental dyslexia: spelling disorders as behavioral phenotypes', *American Journal of Medical Genetics* 67(4), 378–386.

24 A. Boggis (2011), 'Deafening silences: researching with inarticulate children', *Disability and Society* 31(4); T. Booth and W. Booth (1996). 'Sounds of silence: narrative research with inarticulate subjects', *Disability and Society* 18(4), 431–442.

25 S. Firestein (2012). *Ignorance: How It Drives Science*. Oxford: Oxford University Press, p. 92.

26 J. Locke (1689/1975). *An Essay Concerning Human Understanding*. Oxford: Clarendon Press.

27 C. Goodey and M. Rose (2013). 'Mental states, bodily dispositions and table manners: a guide to reading "intellectual" disability from Homer to late antiquity', in C. Laes et al. (eds), *Disabilities in Roman Antiquity: Disparate Bodies*, a Capite ad Calcem. Leiden: Brill.

28 J. Locke (1998). *Two Treatises of Government*. Cambridge: Cambridge University Press.

29 See for example J. Rawls (1971). *A Theory of Justice*. Cambridge, MA: Harvard University Press.

30 Smith, *Being Human*, p. 10.

31 P. Singer (1994). *Rethinking Life and Death: The Collapse of Our Traditional Ethics*. New York: St. Martin's Press.

32 Locke, *An Essay*, p. 571.

33 Moore, *The Formation*.

34 A. Daye (1586/1635). *The Second Part of the English Secretorie*, London: Stansby, p. 235. R. Schalock et al. (2007). 'The renaming of mental retardation: understanding the change to the term intellectual disability', *Intellectual and Developmental Disabilities* 45(2), 116–24.

35 See M. Simpson (2007). 'From savage to citizen: education, colonialism and idiocy', *British Journal of Sociology of Education* 28(5), 561–574. P. McDonagh (2008), *Idiocy: A Cultural History*. Liverpool: Liverpool University Press.

36 T. Gineste (1981). *Victor de l'Aveyron: dernier enfant sauvage, premir enfant fou.* Paris: Sycomore.

37 I am indebted for these points to Patrick McDonagh and Simon Jarrett, whose current work on the transitions towards the institutional era is an advanced state of progress.

38 N. Hervey (1986). 'Advocacy or folly: the Alleged Lunatics' Friend Society, 1845–63', *Medical History* 30, 245–275.

39 P. Bartlett and D. Wright (1999). 'Community care and its antecedents', and J. Walmsley et al. (1999), 'Community care and mental deficiency 1913–1945', in P. Bartlett and D. Wright (eds), *Outside the Walls of the Asylum: The History of Care in the Community 1750–2000.* London: Athlone.

40 See for example P. Ferguson (1994). *Abandoned to Their Fate: Social Policy and Practice toward Severely Retarded People in America, 1820–1920.* Philadelphia, PA: Temple University Press; M. Thomson (1998). *The Problem of Mental Deficiency: Eugenics, Democracy, and Social Policy in Britain c.1870–1959.* Oxford: Oxford University Press; J. Trent (1995). *Inventing the Feeble Mind: A History of Mental Retardation in the United States.* Berkeley: University of California Press; J. Trent and S. Noll (2004). *Mental Retardation in America: A Historical Reader.* New York: New York University Press; D. Wright (2001), *Mental Disability in Victorian England: The Earlswood Asylum.* Oxford: Clarendon.

41 P. McDonagh (2008). *Idiocy: A Cultural History.* Liverpool: Liverpool University Press.

42 See S. Sand (2009). *The Invention of the Jewish People.* London: Verso.

43 R. Moore (2012). *The War on Heresy: Faith and Power in Medieval Europe.* London: Profile Books.

44 M. Burleigh (1994). *Death and Deliverance: Euthanasia in Germany 1900–1945.* Cambridge: Cambridge University Press; G. Aly et al. (1994). *Cleansing the Fatherland: Nazi Medicine and Racial Hygiene.* Baltimore, MD: Johns Hopkins University Press.

5 Causes

The setting is a large consulting room in Harley Street, the epicentre of London's booming private health industry. 'Welcome to our clinic. As single women you are here because you have chosen *not* to bring a child into a relationship that was unsatisfactory. We congratulate you for that. We recommend that you use our donors. The quality of our sperm is two times higher than the national average. With us you simply can't get a dud! We're not creating designer babies [here the salesperson casts a wary side glance at the researcher taking notes] but you want him to be educated and intelligent. You have to be altruistic to donate sperm. You have to be a creative thinker and have a certain level of intelligence. Our student donors are doing a master's or a Ph.D. They come in and donate every week. We get to know them by the coffee machine. If we don't like their personalities, if something doesn't seem right about them – for example, if they don't make eye contact – we don't let them in. We know there are genetic causes of things like autism.'

The banality of the above scenario is reflected at higher levels, in the biological profession itself. David Plotz describes how H. J. Muller, a Nobel prize-winning geneticist, inspired the establishment of a sperm bank of 'genius' reserved for laureates like himself on the basis of their 'intelligence', and of the even vaguer 'outstanding achievements' of a few non-laureate friends.[1] Interwoven with that notion of biological causation lies a mentality plagued with anxiety. The question is, which came first, casual anxiety or causal biology? This problem encapsulates the schizoid nature of inclusion phobia. It has two separate classificatory processes that run in diametrically opposite directions to each other. One can be described by its investigative trajectory, i.e. by what caused the classifier to investigate. It has as its starting-point a social phenomenon, anxiety; this leads to the creation of corresponding psychological subcategories in certain people; these in turn lead to discovery of the natural phenomenon of DNA. The other, by contrast, can be described by its theoretical trajectory. It has as its starting-point a natural phenomenon, DNA; this creates corresponding psychological subcategories; these in turn lead to the social phenomenon of anxiety. The theoretical trajectory, in starting from a permanent fact of nature, obscures the fact that the investigative one took the course it did. In fact the eugenic impulse is both the cause and the product of the biotechnology now available. Seen ahistorically, learning disability constitutes a *motive* – acceptable or unacceptable, according to bioethical taste – for the development of eugenic practices. Seen historically, in all its specificity, it is the conceptual *outcome* of those practices.

Inclusion phobia thus provides an explanation for our explanations. The desire to find a fully scientific explanation for learning disability is a core component of modern biomedical research, and of its funding regimes. Yet the philosophy of science – the monitoring framework, so to speak, for its knowledge claims – regards explanatory claims in biomedicine, especially those that combine elements of the human sciences, as intrinsically incapable of furnishing the necessary precision.[2] For the moment, let's note several respects in which what we take to be facts of the natural world are actually imprecise and transient assumptions, whose specific points of arrival can be tracked in the recent past.

The first is as follows. An *explanation* is not necessarily the same thing as a *cause*. The reduction of the first (the wider term) to the second is typical of modern scientific thinking. In separating knowledge of the body from knowledge of the mind, it proceeds *from* the body *to* the mind. This was not always the case. For example, explanations in ancient medicine, as well as lacking a major conceptual distinction between mind and body, focused on signs rather than causes. Galen, the great Greco-Roman physician of the third century AD who dominated medical discourse up until the eighteenth, placed deficiencies of the mind in the same category and at the same taxonomic level as a long neck or a receding chin. All three were signs of some unsoundness in the material composition of the brain, itself only one of several equally important bodily organs. The explanatory schemes of non-European cultures are of course a different matter again.

The second point connects back to the modernity of the idea of a specifically human intelligence. In Chapter 3, we saw how this is the secularization of intelligence's previous role as a representation of divinity as well as being, conversely, the canonization of a merely human wit that had previously been seen as mundane and nothing special. In parallel with this development, the eighteenth century came up with an increasing preference for one particular argument for the existence of God, out of the several available: the Argument from Design. The two developments gradually became entwined, and modern, atheistic opponents of a creationist Argument from Design – sociobiologists and evolutionary psychologists – are not averse to applying something like it to cognition, intelligence and behaviour.[3] In this respect, the difference between the Christian and the scientific atheist is slim indeed. The ideas of goal-orientation/design and of progress/development towards perfection/ normality lurk in the second group as much as the first, largely through a misinterpretation of the Darwinian principle of evolutionary fitness and its spurious application to the mind.

Learning disability constitutes a crossover point in this respect. In the eighteenth century's religious version of the argument, a natural world whose operations dovetailed in such an orderly way had to have been created by a supremely intelligent being, and to be developing towards a divinely ordained goal. 'Idiots' began to look like a design fault in that picture. Their very existence, as beings seemingly imperfect by creation, appeared to make the religious Argument from Design untenable. Why would a benign God have created them? As non-developmental obstacles to this kind of progress, they contradicted the Argument in principle. These new, positively obstructive 'idiots' helped steer Darwin and his contemporaries *away* from religion.[4] This realization came at exactly the historical point where their 'empirical' existence was being reconstructed in a new, secular guise. Either way, they filled a necessary conceptual space, and perhaps were invented for the purposes of the debate.

The smuggling of the Argument from Design back into evolutionary psychology reflects inclusion phobia's schizoid thought process. The philosopher David Hume was already pointing out in the eighteenth century that you can dismiss God from the Argument from Design without ruling out the idea that the universe tends towards order. In evolutionary psychology, human intelligence and its role in intelligent design are slipped in to replace the Almighty: not only is there order, there is a cognitive goal. With or without religion, notions of intellectual imperfection, deficiency and absence cannot exist without those of perfection. The difference is that today, perfection is chiefly sought in the development of the individual, and only secondarily in that of the species. Ingroup identity now focuses on the development of the individual instead of the Biblical 'lump', and correspondingly on one-by-one elimination of non-developers.

The third creaky floorboard in the edifice of biological causation involves the mind–body split again. As we saw in Chapter 3, the cognitivist vision has roots in medieval philosophy's delusions about the purity of the disembodied soul. Within the last couple of hundred years we have learned to speak the language of mind and body so well that each of the two unavoidably presents itself to us as dependent for its very existence on its separation from the other. However, linking them again, once separated, is problematic. Establishing a *causal* link from one to the other places the problem at a further remove. Saying I have a map of my grandma's genes or my nephew's neurology and that it explains some aspect of their personality is like saying I have a map of Britain and it explains why I have just jumped in my car to visit them. Ask laboratory researchers for examples of a concrete pathway that has been observed leading from one specific gene or complex of genes to one specific cognitive differentiation, even, say, in something as obvious as gender difference, and (to make it easier) if not in humans then in mice. Contrary to what popular science journalists like to hint at, answers beyond the broad brush of chromosomal difference are few. In its account of precise causal detail, cognitive and psychiatric genetics have not progressed much beyond the speculative miasmas of a century ago.

Eugenics and psychological phenotypes

Existing criticisms of eugenics tend to start from the assumption that there is this natural, cross-historical form of difference, learning disability. The nub of the criticism is then, for example, that the 'eugenic impulse' reduces the personhood of such people to some bare physical thing.[5] But the eugenic impulse is more complicated and interesting than that. It is a particularly intense phase of the long shelf-life of inclusion phobia which assumes that *something there must be*, to be bred out. The impulse is prior to any specific target. Tajfel noted this about racism. Social discrimination, he wrote, contributes more to the existence of race than any presumed genetic racial differences in intellectual ability, because those differences 'are already part and parcel of the justifying function of the ideology'.[6] But he neglects to wonder whether the same might not be true for intellectual disability *as such*. The eugenic ideology, as part and parcel of inclusion phobia's classificatory instinct, itself has a causal role: intellectual disability is one of its (temporary) conceptual outcomes. The goal is already embedded in the cause and vice-versa. The very notion of researching causes is value-driven. You would not need to know the cause of something if you did not want to enhance or get rid of it.

Inasmuch as the ingroup now applies the above-mentioned theoretical trajectory to individual bodies, the vague targets of early twentieth-century eugenics *have* been replaced by more scientifically precise testing. Certain experimental possibilities can be made to stick. The more refined the biological causes, the more sharply etched are their associated psychological categories. There is an aggregate of real existences that can be prevented, as a result of biotechnological developments that have followed the investigative trajectory (social anxiety leads to psychological classification leads to biological cause). The cause can then be located empirically within an individual body, with the theoretical trajectory then taking up the thread and leading back to the classification and the exacerbation of the anxiety. And so it goes round.

How do we obtain a fix on a delusion that seems so rational? First, we must isolate the presupposition lurking within the theoretical trajectory. It says that causes operate *from* bodies *to* minds. This presupposition is already a historical contingency. But then comes a further, downright illegitimate step. Biologists typically distinguish between a genotype, the genetic make-up of an organism, and a phenotype, its observable characteristics. Chief among the latter is the somatic phenotype (classically, eye colour or height). Cognitive and behavioural geneticists have extended this theory to the mind, and talk about a psychological or psychiatric phenotype.[7] This step, on which the whole science rests, is no more than an analogy. Insisting on the literal truth of analogies is one strategy in the schizoid screening against reality. From comparing the intangible contents of the mind with material, bodily characteristics, one can jump to the belief that mental or behavioural characteristics belong in the same class of things as bodily ones and that they function similarly in their causal relationship to genes. The opposition between mind and body on which the whole edifice is premised thus collapses in on itself.

This picture of psychological analogies drawn after the event is further contradicted by its own micro-history. The history of science tells us a remarkably clean-limbed story about the Russian monk Gregor Mendel discovering the laws of heredity in peas, but the subsequent detailed application of his discovery in phenotype-genotype theory is a knottier business altogether. It is not the case that biologists started the theory and psychologists took it from there. True, out of this has come the current fashion to classify learning disabilities by their genetic or chromosomal aetiology and thereby to reassign Down's syndrome, for example, to the 'behavioural phenotype' category.[8] And true, it was a biologist who coined the words gene and genotype, and the genotype–phenotype distinction as such. Willem Johannsen's life work was to produce a thoroughbred line of peas, as a way of tracking precise biological laws of heritability; that was why he was then invited on to inter-war Denmark's state commission on degeneracy and eugenics. Here we have the theoretical trajectory, in classic form. But probe his investigatory trajectory, and it runs in the opposite direction. His interest in breeding a pure botanical line was first aroused by reading Galton on the breeding of genius and the differential abilities of the races. It was this, as he himself acknowledged, that inspired him, using the bell curve, to try and create what he called a 'racially pure' line of peas.

Once we situate apparently ahistorical theory in its investigative and historical context, then, we find that its explanations are *from* psychology – and ultimately from anxiety – *to* biology, as well as vice-versa. Both circulate simultaneously, in an alternating current of self-justification. The attempt to eliminate the outgroup is inscribed from the start within the delusional method of classification that cognitive and behavioural phenotypes offer, and within the notion of cause more generally. This does not mean we should be sceptical about biological knowledge as such. It does mean, however, that we need to know the historical context of our current theories and practices.

What are we to make, for example, of the fact that Ernst Rüdin, the pioneer who first proposed an empirical genetic prognosis of psychiatric conditions and thus founded the modern genetics of the mind, would go on to write Nazi Germany's Law on the Prevention of Hereditarily Diseased Offspring, the biological justification for the Holocaust?[9] Can this be viewed as just an ethically warped version of a fundamentally neutral process? Might one not equally suggest a genetic research programme to locate genes for the fabled (when not mythical) affectionateness of people with learning difficulties and to engineer them into the germ line? The reason it sounds unlikely, ethically speaking, is because that supposedly neutral process was itself, historically, the outcome of a more general disorder, inclusion phobia and fear of pollution, in which Rüdin's theory merely forms a specific historical stage. To achieve purity someone must be got rid of. Who?

The ragged edges of the Nazis' category of the hereditarily diseased underline the point. Although an emergent intellectual disability lay at its core, it sucked in the physically disabled and mentally ill too; moreover, the label used for it, 'feeble-minded', encompassed all sorts, as it did everywhere in Europe and America, extending to waifs and strays whose families simply did not want them around any more.

From the perspective of the history of inclusion phobia, it is not ethically shocking, merely appropriate, that Rüdin died at home in bed in 1952 nor even that this was the year when Otmar von Verschuer, Heinrich Himmler's resident eugenicist at Auschwitz and Josef Mengele's academic mentor, would be made Professor of Human Genetics at the University of Münster. I mention them not to illustrate an ethical argument but because the very theoretical basis of the psychiatric and cognitive genetics they dreamed up has been the matrix for everything else – for both the Holocaust and current biotechnological techniques of elimination. The conceptual history of eugenics has a single timespan in which 1945 registers only a blip. This way of looking at that period runs contrary to much of the literature on genetic enhancement, even critical literature, where the basic question seems to be 'Could our biochemical knowledge one day be used to select for intelligence?' when in fact it is already used thus in foetal screening.[10] Ethics in our field can be defined in many cases as the art of finding reasons to eliminate people.

To sum up, the eugenic impulse is the cause *per se* of learning disability as a category, by a process of historical dialectic. Without disability having come to be conceptualized in this way, we would not have had biotechnology itself. If we had not imported the notion of determinism from externals (God, the Devil etc.) to the biology of the individual, the genetics of learning disability would not exist. Today's cognitive and behavioural geneticists complain bitterly about opponents calling them Nazis, as if the falsity of this were self-evident. It may well be false. Name-calling is not a suitable topic on which to pass scientific judgment. What is a matter for science, however, is that geneticists answer for their own discipline, if not for its dubious past then certainly for the destabilising consequences of letting unverifiables such as intelligence and hence learning disability into the laboratory – just as they would have to answer for accidentally letting air into an experiment that needs to be conducted in a vacuum.

Magic and natural causes

In many non-Western or past cultures, causes are not restricted to biology or nature (as we understand it). Cultures ignorant of modern science openly acknowledge a role for magic. This is not to suggest, as Girard at one point tries to do, that magic and scientific method are equivalent and equally contingent. As he himself points out, Claude Lévi-Strauss, in a classic anthropology text, wrote more ambiguously about magical beliefs as 'acts of faith in a science yet to be born'.[11] (This may at least explain why geneticists keep promising a cure for Alzheimer's or Parkinson's, often in return for being allowed to breach existing research ethics guidelines.) Douglas, on the other hand, is content to describe some notions of causality as belonging to 'primitive' societies and others to modern, 'complex' ones. She thinks they are different. But if complex also means scientific, a further distinction is needed. When science claims to explain the causes of thrust reaction in the plane I have just boarded, I am with Douglas. When it claims to explain the causes of intelligence, I am not. The point is: we must recognize the specific limitations of today's scientific method in its *particular field of application*, in our case its application to intelligence and therefore learning disability. It is quite possible that inclusion phobia is not a biological or genetically caused disorder because in its extreme form it seems to belong only in complex societies, though this must remain speculation.

Magic and the supernatural have some relevance at least to present discussions about the causes of learning disability. In another anthropology classic, Mauss referred to magic as 'a gigantic variation on the theme of the principle of causality'.[12] Here, Girard's relativist polemic does become pertinent: 'Magical thought does not originate in disinterested curiosity. It is usually the last resort in a time of [looming] disaster, and provides principally a system of accusation ... at the level of social relations.'[13] The resonance with modern explanations for learning disability is that both are symptoms of a social paranoia whose roots lie in fear of the Devil. His malign influence on our social world was thought by the early Royal Society to come not through the *super*natural but through his skilful and lightning-quick manipulation of existing nature, known as 'natural magic' (Boyle's interest in the laws of chemistry sprang from this idea).[14]

Here, then, is the appropriate point to discuss 'nature versus nurture', where nature is assumed to be more or less deterministic. First of all, it should be noted that most binary formulae are ways of closing down discussion. The fact that there can only be one thing or the other, another example of 'splitting', is a structural expression of inclusion phobia. Regardless of whether nature and nurture interact or not, the formula implies that there are some things nurture cannot touch. Learning disability fulfils that role. In this debate determinism is thought of as characteristic of nature as such, but beneath this lies a prior thought: that natural causes are determinate *because determinateness is something that is by definition beyond our reach*. It implies that we cannot know about any causal link further back in the chain from nature except for a *super*natural one. Thus the nature–nurture formula is pure metaphysics and not worth taking sides over.

The idea of nature as a deterministic type of cause is in fact the modern reduction of an earlier formula that was three-way, between nature, nurture and necessity, rather than two-way. In this medieval obsession with threes (derived from the Christian doctrine of the Trinity) nature meant something closer to what today we call second nature, and lay between nurture and necessity. Before the modern era, people's very social position depended on an interplay between 'ability' – a mixture of economic, social and psychological elements – and their 'disposition'; determinism lay elsewhere, as we shall see. And it was disposition that constituted human nature. When the doyen of medieval philosophers Albert the Great wrote about people who are 'stupid from birth' (again, he would have probably included most of the population in this), it signified chiefly their disposition.[15] How people were 'trained-up' or 'inured' overlapped both nature and nurture in their modern senses.[16] Robert Burton's ubiquitous *The Anatomy of Melancholy*, a kind of seventeenth-century DSM, defines nature in human beings as the 'whole manner of living' and 'continual practices', shaped by 'the country or soil wherein one is born'. And when he calls 'intelligence' a 'natural' phenomenon, he says explicitly that he means by this word a 'habit' or disposition.[17] Human nature, as such, is not innate. Everything apart from conscience, a divine spark slipped in by God, is dispositional. God created the 'rational soul' or mind equal in every human embryo; intellectual and behavioural differences were caused by something less essential.

Determinism lay neither in nature nor in nurture but in what was eventually called 'necessity', whose precursor notions were religious (predestination) and social (fate). Thus there was not a dyad but a triad. Galton's formula 'nature vs nurture' now dominates possibly because he introduced statistics into the discussion; primitive statistics found it easier to deal with two variables than with three. At any rate, we can safely ignore his claim to have got it from Shakespeare, who had used the pairing in a quite different way. Nevertheless, one of Shakespeare's contemporaries was indeed just starting to endow nature with deterministic properties, as scientific method began to engage with the physical world. Historians of science have seen a connection between this attempt to know and control nature and the Stuart monarchy's aim to control its subjects. Where the mind is concerned, the connection is more than mere parallelism. After all, at the peak moment of absolutism in English political history, the inventor of scientific method and James I's Lord Chancellor turn out to have been the same person. The call by Francis Bacon, a.k.a. Lord Verulam, for an experimental basis to physics and chemistry sparked a process in which *human* nature itself would become no longer a disposition or 'code of behaviour so much as the most vital of human resources: one utilised by an intellectual elite, under the authority of the state, for the common good'.[18]

The fact that the nature of the mind too was starting to be a less floppy concept suggested to political authority new prospects for controlling its subjects and above all for controlling their suspect *inner* states. By the end of the nineteenth century it would be clear that this could be achieved not only by tighter classification of those states but even better, in cases of anomaly and abnormality, by a eugenic rooting out their material causes and of the individual people who embodied them.

Normal/abnormal is another reduction of a formerly three-way scheme: natural/unnatural/praeternatural. Before the modern era, any individuals described as unnatural were in the last resort exotic specimens of the natural; monsters tended to belong in nature, not outside it. They were accidents – a term used in logic to mean some oddity that did not contradict membership of a category. Whatever these accidental individuals' deficiencies, they were still fully paid-up members of the species. The word praeternatural, by contrast, was used for causes that lay outside the human realm altogether. In Greek and Roman medicine this had meant the environment; in Christianity, it meant either God or the Devil, chiefly the latter. Praeternatural causes were close to the deterministic idea of necessity, but in this case with diabolic over-tones. With the triad reduced to a pairing, the difference between unnatural and praeternatural was lost; encouraged by the rise of statistics, they combined to form what we now know as the abnormal – a more watertight version of the extreme outgroup.

The Devil as the cause of learning disability

Two major misunderstandings about the Devil hamper our historical under-standing of intelligence. First, that the arrival of modern science put an end to belief in the Devil as the cause of things that go wrong; second, that belief in the Devil was a superstition of laypeople and the masses, which knowledge elites sought to cure them of. Removing these misunderstandings will show how inclusion phobia and the new formulae about biological cause were involved in the very creation of learning disability as we know it today.

The modern psychology of intelligence, at least in its divisive classificatory tendencies, is the phoenix that arose from the ashes of election and repro-bation theory. Reprobates had existed *en masse*. All human beings were reprobate through Adam's fall. The elect, with their receptivity to grace, were simply reprobates whom God had graciously decided to save; everyone else was still shackled to the Devil. The elect were supposedly a very small ingroup indeed, though many more liked to think of themselves as members.[19] Once the seventeenth century's fanatical wars of religion (among other things) were over, the doctrine of instantly *conferred* grace in the few was replaced by the more sober idea that one should use one's reason, as a means to *achieve* grace. It caused aspiration to expand, aided by education. Although the mid-seventeenth-century demise of predestination theory was very sudden, the sublimation of reprobates within the new type of extreme outgroup took a long time to play out.

Increased optimism about elect status corresponded with the gradual reduction of the corresponding outgroup to a small minority. A common symptom of inclusion phobia is that the smaller the extreme group that is the focus of its paranoid attentions, the greater the threat it poses. There was thus a much greater urgency to the question of what causes such creatures to be born. While there were also theories which said that God created them as 'innocents' free from sin, and other theories that already regarded nature as a neutral force, the Devil retained a presence, all the more potent for being less talked about. In the old predestination doctrine reprobates had merely enlis-ted on the Devil's side, and the Devil's natural powers were subordinate to God's. On the threshold of the modern era, the Devil's supposed ability to intervene in procreation meant his stature was increasing.

Old doctrines were being replaced not only by a greater anxiety about causes but also, with respect to disability, by the idea that certain diabolic causes might lie within the parents. The novel idea of the Devil as a creator or co-creator of outgroup individuals, along with their increasingly pathological identity, solved the problem about God being the author of their imperfection, but on top of this was a new story about class which, rather than ditching the old one, adjusted it to a changing social context. It came not from conservatives or reactionaries but from forward-looking radical democrats such as the Levellers, and from the founders of political liberalism.

When Locke, for example, writes about idiots, he says that they lack the skills of abstraction and logical reasoning. But the word idiot was by now ambiguous. He may still be using the word in its class sense, as the medieval clerical caste had done. On the other hand, in his new account of our reasoning operations, the 'abstracting' skills which idiots lacked are already a universal human characteristic. He also refers, in the same work, to 'changelings'. It is not clear whether his idiots are idiots in the old class sense or equivalent to these genuinely pathological creatures upon whom the whole weight of the fear of animality is projected. The two terms seem in the end to be scarcely distinguishable; moreover he uses 'natural fool' as a synonym for both. Be that as it may, his discussion of causes was rooted in religion as well as (more or less indistinguishably) in politics, and directly influenced the modern concept of learning disability. In religious terms, the idea of a changeling child evoked the theory that newborns might be replaced in the cradle by witches, or that a demonic incubus had impregnated the mother. In social, genealogical terms, it might mean a false heir. Exactly as Locke sweated over the last few pages of his pioneering texts on empirical psychology and political liberalism, a national debate about a 'changeling' of another type was taking place. It attended the unexpected and scandalous birth of a son to James II's menopausal wife, a wrong child if ever there was one because it meant the next monarch would be a Catholic like his despised father (he would later feature as The Old Pretender).

Once the mid-century religious and political wars had stopped, and with them the controversies over election and reprobation, it became in retrospect dangerous or at least impolite to talk of the Devil. As belief in the Devil went underground, his subliminal presence in the modern mindset increased. The new Royal Society experimentalists such as Boyle, Newton and Locke himself, took his existence very seriously and tried to work out how he intervenes in natural processes, including biological ones. Here, on the threshold of the modern era, the idea that the Devil had a role in producing disabled children was spreading in scientific circles, not receding. Similar origins can be discerned in bioethics. If some maintain that there is a minority whose lack of genetically determined cognitive skills means their human status is questionable and euthanasia justifiable, that is directly because religious thinkers once maintained that there are reprobate 'monsters' whose 'seminal' or divinely determined lack of a rational religion meant that they were not in grace. Singer's position on euthanasia for people like this is an echo of John Bunyan's warning that reprobates 'must perish for their unreasonableness'.[20]

Modern and pre- or early modern theoretical trajectories may differ, with DNA replacing the Devil, but they share a metaphysical element, that of necessity and determinism. At the level of social history, the differing histor-ical trajectories have in common the banality we observed at the start of this chapter. Take a key development such as the clear distinction between intel-lectual disability and mental illness. What could sound more like scientifically grounded theory? In fact this tightened codification of human types and behaviours was part of a more general move in the English language towards precise referents in this period. The particular terms of the codification arose from cultural jousting among members of the literary elite in the 1590s. The Tudor monarchs had been reviving, for fiscal purposes, an obscure medieval distinction that bore only the loosest connection to any condition we might recognize today. When writers and poets used the 'idiot or lunatic?' formula, it was to insult each other, not a differential diagnosis. This new terminology nevertheless fed into medico-legal classifications of incompetence over the next century, simply by its availability. In the investigative trajectory of psy-chiatric classification, then, the language of insult could be said to have as much of a causative role as biology.

Something similar happened with the institutions. Just as the role of the Devil in generating (modern) idiots *began* at the same time as modern science, so too did the practice of visiting Bedlam to be entertained. An obsessive preoccupation with *types* of madness (Locke's 'several ways of faltering') developed, a pathological behaviour in which laughter was part of the mix. The origin of this interest was not medical at all. Bethlehem Hospital itself had always run a recognisably therapeutic, if austere, regime. Instead, it was the ubiquitous stage *mis*representations of Bedlam, from the Jacobean play-wrights onwards, that inspired the gentry to visit the place as observers, and this fed into precursor forms of psychiatric classification.[21] They laughed in the hospital because they had laughed in the theatre. A classic example for our purposes is Middleton and Rowley's *The Changeling*. In 1622 this word had denoted someone who kept changing their mind, as several of the play's main characters do – though the play does also feature someone who disguises himself as a fool of the 'idiot' type in order to seduce the asylum-keeper's wife. Half a century later the study of human behaviour had sidelined the will by comparison with human reason. The 'changeling' label may in the interim have got subconsciously transferred from a pathology of the will to one of intelligence; people's recollection of the wilful main characters got mixed up with that of the fake fool. This confusion then enabled the classification process to take the course it did.

The child you have had or the child you haven't had?

Like the theologian, the average medieval peasant too may have invoked the Devil, but probably in trivial ways. If he got up in the morning to find his breakfast loaf half eaten, he might mutter 'What the Devil ...' but the poor idiot would mainly be thinking he had a problem with mice. Theologians, experts on the mind among other things, knew better, and relied increasingly on the Devil to explain the social world around them. The peasant only had to get on with satisfying his croaking belly, whereas the theologian needed to sit around all day worrying about why bad things happen. Belief in the praeternatural, and some knowledge of how it worked, was a guarantee of their authenticity as thinkers, and their membership of a knowledge elite. When Hieronymus Bosch depicted devils he was not merely using folk imagery for rhetorical effect, he was indoctrinating the congregation: 'You'd better believe it.' The Reformation subsequently built an intellectual apparatus around the Devil to explain our disastrous lives on earth. They also democratized that belief. The result was that now 'Men and women of the world were glad, // Who'd never cared or trembled in their lives'.[22] That was how, from the mid-seventeenth century onward, he became sublimated within our understandings of the social realm.

The key to the sublimation process lay in utilitarianism: the idea that the solution to social and ethical problems should focus on the consequences of our actions and the maximization of utility (the greatest happiness). It is possible to see how this might fit a statistical, quantitative and assessment-based mentality, but more difficult to see in what sense it was/is a religious one. After all Jeremy Bentham, its supposed inventor (in fact its modernizer), was notoriously an atheist. The new focus on moral consequences replaced one in which the solution to problems of right and wrong had been sought in the heart and intentions of the believer. So how does the Devil still thrive at the core of today's mainstream, atheistic doctrine? Theological contemporaries of Bentham had injected a toxic dose of utilitarianism into the Argument from Design.[23] The ultimate purpose of the design was for God to promote happiness: a perfection not only of the natural order but also of the social order. Imperfection in certain individuals, once just part of the warp and weft of nature, was a direct threat to society conceived in these new progressivist terms, regardless of whether the terms were religious or not.

Utilitarianism has been a central value in the elimination practices of the twentieth and twenty-first centuries. The main debating point among historians of the Nazi euthanasia programme is about whether its aim was utilitarian in the sense of the reduction of fiscal expenditure (which is how it was first presented to the German people) or ideological (the acting out of social Darwinism). But an understanding of the historical evolution of inclusion phobia in its concrete totality shows that both aims amount to the same thing. In its apparently secular guise utilitarianism is a core principle, inasmuch as pre-natal testing saves public money that would otherwise have to be spent on disabled people (though this is spurious, as segregation is more expensive than support for ordinary lives) – when actually the very concept 'intellectually disabled people', let alone the urge to eliminate them, is predicated on the schizoid delusions of its religious roots.

Utilitarianism, both religious and atheistic, was a corollary to the new medical and biological emphasis on causes. Causes imply consequences. And the more the consequences were about developmental progress towards some earthly perfection rather than the afterlife, the greater the room for identifying hindrances, and for rooting them out along with their causes. Major natural disasters of the early eighteenth century helped to reinforce the Devil's sub-liminal presence in the minds of ordinary people too. They were cured of their short-sightedness in seeing bad events as temporary social dislocations and inoculated with a phobic belief that there were underlying causes mediated by unnatural individuals, whose malign influence was self-evident in their deficiencies.[24]

In cases where diagnosis is made at birth or early infancy, a direct line runs from then till now. Popular culture – or so it seems – imputes to parents the idea that they have had a different child from the one they expected. In fact it is a hand-me-down from the proto-psychiatric knowledge elites of an earlier era; they are themselves the source of that superstitious attitude towards the child, which they attribute to their lay parental inferiors via the bereavement analogy. The idea that sperm or newborn infants could be swapped or that there was an original child who is now missing comes not from folklore but from experts on human behaviour. In twenty-first-century London, as witch-doctors in immigrant communities are accused of conducting ritual child abuse by telling parents that their children turn into cats or dogs at night, profes-sionals are counselling the parents of infants newly diagnosed with learning disability to 'grieve for the child they have not had'.[25] Meanwhile the suppo-sedly primitive cruelty which West African village communities are alleged to mete out to children with learning difficulties, whom they see as 'snake children', invites comparison with an advanced technology preoccupied with eliminating snake embryos.[26]

Such are the rituals by which inclusion phobia is projected and displaced onto a lay population. This is one case where distinctions within the ingroup have to be maintained. And so ritual is clothed in science. Parental reactions are pathologized as much as the disability. Viewed through the psychiatric lens of coping theory, which describes reactions to shock, they are said to undergo a strict list of stages of acceptance of the infant, and of symptoms that start with denial (to be followed by rejection, anger, etc.). However, the idea that this is not the child you actually conceived was to start with the knowledge elite's *own* theory about the cause of deficiency. Such elites, whe-ther theological or psychiatric, have elements of a continuous profile, and when modern elites attribute to others the idea that this is not the real child, they are projecting on to parents some equally paranoid thought processes of their own. Parents whose children have been diagnosed at birth have some-times reported being asked by doctors and nurses if they are planning to have another – an appropriate moment to be receiving the question, since it clearly means (as one parent paraphrased it) 'Go away and have a real one'.

How does the schizoid denial of history cope with historical shifts that are so big they are unmissable? It seems that when knowledge elites move on to a new causal paradigm, they deal with their embarrassment at having subscribed to the stupid one they now reject by attributing it to the ignorant masses instead. It becomes 'superstition'. The existence of superstition is itself then made scientific by crediting it with natural status; the bereavement analogy and the idea that this is not my child are something a parent thinks 'naturally'. This reification of the changeling story – a lingering echo of an era when the idiot outgroup was the whole lay public – can be traced seamlessly from its seventeenth-century theological origins via the Brothers Grimm and thence into twenty-first-century psychiatry.[27]

This is not to deny that parents often repeat the analogy, in a feedback effect from the negative story handed down by elites. It has been adopted by large voluntary organizations. The result is that parents who love their children as they are may also make much of their difficulties because that is what the world seems to expect of them. Genuine distress, by contrast, is caused less by the child, less even than by having to get up three times a night, than by the inclusion phobia of the world beyond the family. And it is probably rare for professionals to have said something about overall patterns of a particular learning disability (as distinct from common-sense advice about discrete behaviours) that has led a family to behave differently towards their child, or in such a way as to endorse the idea of bereavement.

The bereavement analogy and its highlighting of the causes of difference is a picturesque image that may help with fund-raising (though usually not for any kind of intervention that might extend the ordinariness of the parent–child relationship to that of the social institutions beyond it). A sunnier version, currently popular, runs: 'I booked a week in Venice, there was a problem with the flights and I ended up holidaying in Belgium – but Belgium's quite a nice place when you get to know it'. It still begs the question why I was expecting, before my child was born, to land in one place rather than any other. It was because I already had modern psychology's map, with its idea of perfection as normality, in my head.

There is also contrary and more positive sociological evidence to show that families expand their concept of the normal to include the new arrival; if there is acceptance, it is not of the child's disability but of its full humanity.[28] In that case there seems no need for an alternative view on what caused it, or any view at all. The stress reported by parents, when examined microscopically, seems to involve battling to understand precisely that they do not share the world view of the person imparting the diagnosis; or they will often report the event as having changed themselves and their lives for the better.[29] However, these studies rely on qualitative methodologies involving in-depth interviews, whose status as valid research is increasingly ignored and denied both by the clinic and by government. Families who expand the boundaries of the normal expect other social institutions outside, as they draw individuals away from family networks, to do the same, and they do not. Some families accept this situation (yet another meaning of that word acceptance), others perceive the irrationality of the system that excludes a family member and of the person who does the excluding.

Approaches can be ambiguous. Social constructionists, as we have already noted, tend to hang out with both gangs at once. Entirely positive things such as parental love are said to be motives for an equally positive urge to emphasize difference.[30] Alternatively, if normal parenting is itself a social construction, it cannot be there to be expanded and families 'perform' a constructed normality instead. On the one hand, they do not consider the child alien to them; on the other, the implication remains that they are making the best of a bad job.[31] The badness can of course only be the disability. Such approaches, whatever else they do, also reinforce the phobia. So too does the labelling by Frith and others of parents as heroes.[32] The implication is that what is *normal* is *not* to accept the child ('The gist: parents are heroes if they do not reject their children'[33]). And when parents do play the heroic role, it certainly *is* only a performance, often conducted for the purpose of obtaining support. Status is a zero sum: if credit accrues to some people, it can only be by debiting others.

Parental guilt

Causes involve parents in another way. In early Christianity, the prevailing view was that God created the human soul – the 'rational soul' – and infused it in the embryo some weeks after conception. This soul was an attribute of everyone by virtue of their membership of the species. Its presence was a sign of the equality of all human creatures. It did not require assessment, and as God's creation it certainly could not be subject to deficiency. The lay masses may have been stupid by disposition, but their souls were as sound as the cleverest philosopher's. However, there had always been a rival theory, which claimed that the soul arrived at conception, by natural generation from the parents.

A minority view to begin with, by the mid-seventeenth century it was providing serious competition. The debate about it threw up compromise versions in which God and the parents were joint providers. Parental participation in the creation of the soul could explain better why some people were *so* deficient, at a time when extreme outgroup deficiency was just beginning to be theorized. And it led to the concept of other partners too – not only praeternatural or demonic ones but animals (in which case the child was only half-rational), or same-sex ones. All these possible causes placed offspring within the realm of the unnatural, which by now was acquiring a praeternatural twist. The Leveller democrat Richard Overton saw such children ('buggery births', as he termed them) not as the product of nature but of 'God's curse', and as entirely lacking a rational soul. Locke clearly thought something similar about the cause of 'changeling' children, though his starched prurience prevented him from being explicit about it.

Here are the roots of several nineteenth-century ideas that coincide with the formal arrival of the psychology of intelligence and disability. Its distinction between imbeciles and idiots, still going strong in our 'moderate' and 'severe', can be traced back to people like Overton who drew a line within the outgroup by ascribing different causative agencies (natural in the case of the former, praeternatural in the latter), or to Locke and his distinction between idiots and changelings. Meanwhile the link from learning disability to sexuality had become trivialized, as supposed sexual deviance; the pioneering American educator Samuel Gridley Howe, for example, thought it was caused by parents who masturbated.

Nevertheless, these ideas remained elite and theoretical, unrelated to actual social history. Parents of any social class rarely read such obscure stuff. In fact the history of parental guilt is much more recent. It only took hold once the long-stay institutions began to give certain people a much sharper profile by distancing them geographically from their communities. The second half of the twentieth century would then be preoccupied with expunging the guilt feelings. The most spectacular example of the modern exculpation of parents comes with autism, which in the immediate post-war era was attributed to 'refrigerator mothers' but now produces those heroes who stand at the opposite deviation from the norm. Just as the eugenic impulse was not only a response to the existence of learning disability but also a cause of its conceptualization, so the history of parental guilt and its removal are not just reactions to the disability but themselves have had a causative role in the establishment, prolongation and passing of the concept. Following the brief historical span – a century at most – in which parents were made (or more likely assumed) to feel guilty, they have dropped out completely from the frame of investigation into the causes of evil. They and their biology are now value-free. However, this impacts the evil, the negative value, entirely onto the DNA and therefore onto the child itself. The driver of this infernal machine is the paranoid beliefs of inclusion phobia.

Notes

1 D. Plotz (2005). *The Genius Factory: The Curious History of the Nobel Prize Sperm Bank*. New York: Random House.
2 P. Kitcher (1989). 'Explanatory unification and the causal structure of the world', in P. Kitcher and W. Salmon, *Scientific Explanation*. Minneapolis: University of Minnesota Press, pp. 410–505.
3 P. Griffiths, 'Dancing in the dark: evolutionary psychology and the argument from design', in S. Scher and F. Rauscher (2012). *Evolutionary Psychology: Alternative Approaches*. New York: Springer.
4 F. Darwin (1887). *The Life and Letters of Charles Darwin, Including an Autobiographical Chapter*. London: John Murray, ii, p. 311.
5 G. Agamben (1998). *Homo Sacer: Sovereign Power and Bare Life*. Stanford, CA: Stanford University Press.
6 Tajfel, *Human Groups*, p. 38.
7 R. Dawkins (1989). *The Extended Phenotype*. Oxford: Oxford University Press; M. Leboyer et al. (1998), 'Psychiatric genetics: search for phenotypes', *Trends in Neurosciences* 21(3), 102–105.
8 See for example D. Skuse (2000). 'Behavioural phenotypes: what do they teach us?' *Archives of Disease in Childhood* 82, 222–225.
9 See J. Joseph and N. Wetzel (2013). 'Ernst Rüdin: Hitler's racial hygiene mastermind', *Journal for the History of Biology* 46(1), 1–30.
10 D. Kirby (2000). 'The new eugenics in cinema: genetic determinism and gene therapy in *Gattaca*', *Science Fiction Studies* 27(2), 193–215.

11 Girard, *The Scapegoat*, p. 52.
12 Cited in Girard, p. 52.
13 Girard, p. 53.
14 S. Shapin and S. Schaffer (1994). *A Social History of Truth: Civility and Science in Seventeenth-Century England*. Chicago: University of Chicago Press.
15 Albertus Magnus, *Ethica* I.47, in *Albertus Magnus: Works Online*. www.alber tusmagnus.uwaterloo.ca
16 Daye, *The Second Part*, p. 236.
17 R. Burton (1621/1973). *The Anatomy of Melancholy*, vol. 1. Littlehampton: Everyman's University Library.
18 P. Withington (2005). *The Politics of Commonwealth: Citizens and Freemen in Early Modern England*. Cambridge: Cambridge University Press, p. 54.
19 See Chapter 4.
20 J. Bunyan (1674). *Reprobation Asserted*. London: G.L.
21 C. Neely (2004). *Distracted Subjects: Madness and Gender in Shakespeare and Early Modern Culture*. Ithaca, NY: Cornell University Press.
22 W. H. Auden (1976). 'Luther', in *Collected Poems* (ed. E. Mendelson). London: Faber.
23 F. Rosen (2003). *Classical Utilitarianism from Hume to Mill*. London: Routledge.
24 See R. Fenn (1995). *The Persistence of Purgatory*. Cambridge: Cambridge University Press.
25 J. Davenport, 'Warning as number of witchcraft child abuse cases rise in London', *London Evening Standard*, 9 October 2014.
26 M. Bayat (2015). 'The stories of "snake children": the killing and abuse of children with developmental disabilities in West Africa', *Journal of Intellectual Disability Research* 59(1), 1–10.
27 C. Goodey and T. Stainton (2001), 'Intellectual disability and the myth of the changeling myth', *Journal for the History of the Behavioural Sciences* 37(3), 223–240.
28 T. Booth (1978). 'From normal baby to handicapped child', *Sociology* 12, 203–221.
29 See for example T. Stainton and H. Besser (1998). 'The positive impact of children with an intellectual disability on the family', *Journal of Intellectual and Developmental Disability* 23, 57–70; P. Fisher and D. Goodley (2007). 'The linear medical model of disability: mothers of disabled babies resist', *Sociology of Health and Illness* 29(1), 66–81.
30 C. Silverman (2013). *Understanding Autism: Parents, Doctors, and the History of a Disorder*. Princeton, NJ: Princeton University Press; A. Solomon (2014). *Far from the Tree: Parents, Children and the Search for Identity*. New York: Vintage.
31 M. Voysey (1975/2006). *A Constant Burden: The Reconstitution of Family Life*. Farnham: Ashgate.
32 B. Firestone (2007). *Autism Heroes: Portraits of Families Meeting the Challenge*. London: Jessica Kingsley.
33 Easter Seals Disability Services, Chicago. http://blog.easterseals.com/are-parents-of-children-with-autism-heroes. Retrieved 27 December 2014.

6 Development

Sophie laughs, showing that she likes the company of some people more than others, and the people she does enjoy she enjoys each in their different way. She wears a bib with her school uniform and it is getting wet; someone is going to come and change it, and check her posture (a strap holds her in her wheelchair). Everyone has agreed that this is better than her wearing some medical overall. 'It's just who she is', the class teacher tells me. The other students interact normally with her because they know that communication is not just about speech or sight (she does not use words or see). They are learning about geology, and Sophie has some rocks to feel. She is part of the fabric of this academically successful comprehensive school in East London; among the students she is sitting alongside are future doctors, lawyers and psychologists. By any cognitive test she does not reach 'stages'. Does she perceive herself as having developmental goals, for which her intelligence will be the crucial lever? Should she?

This begs a prior question. What is more essentially human about Sophie: is it that she belongs in the world with others? Or is it some form of rationality and intelligence that she may or may not develop? This sets two fundamental traditions of Western thought in opposition to each other. Although the question might seem purely philosophical, real life comes into it. First of all, there is the fact that Sophie is there at all, belying the phobic assumption in most discussions about education that there must always be *someone* who cannot be included, and that if an example were needed then Sophie would be it. Second, there is historical evidence. No one before the modern era had a concept of psychological development, or of developmental intelligence in particular.

The historical contingency of the idea of psychological development, and the specifically modern socio-economic roots and motives which gave rise to it, are clear enough. 'Development' developed. Human cultures of the distant past situated the life of an individual more in space than in time. Today's emphasis on time seems lop-sided in the context of this longer historical perspective. Moreover, development is only one possible way of describing how time passes in the individual person. It is culturally constructed so as to help us make sense of ourselves, to each other and about each other, at this particular conjuncture. It corresponds to the move away from time as seasonal and cyclical, typical of agricultural communities, and towards something that is goal-oriented, commodified and measurable. It is true that in pre-modern agricultural economies childhood may have been an investment in the provision of external support for the future or for the continuation of landholding. Nevertheless that future consisted of repeated cycles. Without a linear, non-cyclical notion of societal progress, there was no need to internalize development within the inner nature of individuals.

If we want to understand what cognitive development truly is, we must (as with intelligence itself) shed the carapace of received wisdom and look at its historical onset, as a concept. Its role in inclusion phobia represents a particular phase in the economic, political and social history of Western Europe. What are its essential characteristics?

First of all, as with the teleological argument for the existence of God, this idea that human beings develop signifies that a *goal* is already inscribed at the beginning of the path leading towards it. Cognitive development develops towards what you have already decided you will find. Piaget, for example, writes about development in terms of 'mental logic', seen as a form of intellectual perfection (read: normality) that is the ultimate stage of human existence. Yet development only takes the form it does, or any form at all, because he and many of the rest of us have already decided, within the relatively recent past, on a goal of earthly perfection, that the goal is indeed achievable, and that this – in the form of normal intelligence and above – is what it is. Perfection of the species is normality in the individual. Development fits accordingly. And abnormality consists in not developing. Some such picture is at the core of a seemingly optimistic developmentalism like Vygotsky's as much as of Piaget's rigidly structural account.

Second, goals entail *progress*: some idea about how to get from where you are now to where you want to be. This may seem obvious, but it was not always the case. Aristotle too had a teleological view of human nature and social goals, but it was static, not temporal. The nature of the human individual, he said, was to live in a natural community: it was community that was the goal. All conceivable types of exception to this rule – the mad, the uncivilized, wild men of the woods – he included within it. Later on the Renaissance was full of writers noting superficially how 'the child becomes the man', but this did not involve the concept of a temporal development of the individual's inner life, only some vague aspirations about their moral virtue. In modern developmental psychology, by contrast, it just goes without saying that there is an intellectual goal-directedness within the individual that plays out over time; its importance to the community is signalled by the fact that exceptional types – those in whom that goal-directedness is absent – are now a hindrance. Hence their elimination is a priority for the public funding of biomedical research.

Third, though, if everyone reached perfection, why would we need developmental psychology? The answer is that it exists to maintain a gradient of superiority/inferiority even within the ingroup band of normal. This is necessary to avoid the crisis of differentiation. The purpose of ejecting and persecuting an extreme outgroup is to guarantee the existence of status differentials within the ingroup. That is the non-developing outgroup's raison d'être, it *is* nothing else. The concept of development expresses the increasing sharpness with which inclusion phobia has delineated human groups over the last couple of centuries. The thought process is, again, schizoid. The education of students like Sophie is tested in UK schools by *p* scales. *p* comes before level 1. Does it belong to the general system, then, or doesn't it? It clearly aims to be both. *p* stands for performance, but actually it is non-performance. In practice the very notion of a scale is irrelevant to some students; but the *p* scale has to exist in theory because the system says levels in general have to exist. Thus its reason for existence is to reinforce the validity of having levels 1 and above within the ingroup.

Developmental disability and the nature of childhood

The nakedly schizoid character of inclusion phobia is evident above all where children are involved. Even in the few countries where the policy aspiration for adults with learning difficulties is that they lead ordinary lives in the community, children are effectively exempt from the principle. Despite educational legislation that makes a pious nod to the inclusive principle, they are effectively barred from ordinary schools. It is a self-preserving system; families, while not endorsing special schools with any enthusiasm, are mostly unaware of the possibilities that Sophie and her classmates have. Any general political commitment to inclusion will always evoke exclusion as its binary partner, affirming the latter by handing it an unwarranted cachet of sanity.[1] The UK Equalities and Human Rights Commission, for example, in the same breath as endorsing the unconditional commitment in the UN Convention on the Rights of Disabled Persons to inclusive education, warns that for 'children with very severe learning difficulties … this is neither possible nor appropriate'.[2] The only logical way out of this contradiction is to say that they are not actually human or (to use Locke's words) do not have a soul.

So much for the rights of people with learning difficulties. In practice and politics, the categorization of learning disability and that of childhood in general are closely intertwined. Here is another illustration. Having been involved in researching the closure of segregated schools in one London borough, I went to speak about what had been happening to a meeting in another borough, which had had success in tackling disability discrimination and meeting the government's targets for adult employment (mostly for physically disabled people) but whose levels of school segregation remained high. I arrived assuming that the audience would already be with me, but soon realized my mistake. There was a reaction that seemed like opposition, but above all an air of puzzlement. What on earth did this have to do with *them*? What was the connection between employment rights and abolishing segregation? It took some minutes before the penny dropped: ah, you're talking about *children*. Following a rights-based line, the link they saw was one between the right of adults to employment and the right of adult teachers to exclude (especially in cases of severe learning disability and 'behavioural disorder'). Nevertheless, the misunderstanding lay deeper. The notion of rights did not apply to children: that is – this meant not just disabled children but all children. How could this audience have understood the intrinsic parallel between inclusive education and inclusive employment without first accepting that children *in general* are already fully human?

Modern notions of childhood are predicated on those of development. Before the modern era, a child was an undersized adult. Today, to be a child is effectively to be intellectually disabled – an identity imposed on children by the idea that certain creatures exist who have not reached a potential perfection.[3] In the same way that difference as learning disability overlaps with difference by class, gender or race, so difference as developmental disability overlaps with difference by age. The very idea of development is an instrument for the repression of children, who within modern forms of social organization are among those people who sometimes need more support than others. Just as development is today's idea, the past, in lacking a notion of cognitive disability, also lacked today's notion of childhood in general.

Developmental theories are formed from normative definitions of childhood of which *stages* are the building blocks. Stages suggest markers (has this child reached stage *x* and when will it do so?), which lead in turn to the idea that the child can be assessed on the basis of 'observation' (in a sense that mimics the hard sciences' use of the term). Sociologists have seen competence in terms of shifting and contingent social experiences rather than of assessment, and childhood itself as a non-existent concept in some eras and cultures.[4] We can go further. The modern category of the child, especially in its developmental sense, is another projection of inclusion phobia. However, children are not an extreme outgroup like the intellectually disabled because the vast majority have a ticket dated for some future point of entry. They are candidate members of the ingroup. Following the sixteenth-century religious origins of this view of children, they have been seen as in a state of becoming rather than being, that is, of becoming intellectually mature adults. Children, then, are idiots – but temporary ones.

Without this modern concept of childhood as chronological deficiency, and of learning disability as the failure to emerge from it, we could not have the concept of development as such. To have intellectually disabled people, we must have modern children, and vice-versa. The whole idea of development is founded on difference, in this case the difference between adults' normal cognitive processes and the incomplete ones of children. Modern disabled people are routinely seen as childish or at best childlike; and without our own historically specific concept of childhood we could not see disability as a developmental plateau.

Psychological *development* is partly modelled on economic *investment*, and assessment on accounting procedures. However, it is not just that current educational ideologies promote the construction, via normal cognitive processes, of an economically competent individual who will contribute to the growth of international capital. The developmental and the economic belong in each other's delusions. The teacher is required to invest in a child's development, as you would invest money in a slot machine and expect chocolate to come out. If it doesn't, you may kick it hopefully or call in a specialist to try and fix it, and if it still doesn't work, the machine is taken away and dumped in a separate space at the back with all the other dud machines. The psychopathic element in this particular trait of inclusion phobia is the removal of certain people from normal everyday circulation, while also indicating the wider psychopathy of treating children in general as machines for exploitation.

The idea of development belongs in inclusion phobia's dream of its own permanence. Its virus-like aim of adapting in order to live forever makes for a tense relationship between the spatial and the temporal. In one sense developmentalism is a temporal concept, an internal reflection of social progress within the individual. In another way it 'denies history' in Gabel's sense, inasmuch as it blanks out any notion of a time when people did not have a concept of development. But be that as it may, it does not deny itself a glorious future. From the restricted standpoint of its own social niche in the intelligence society, it has a goal firmly in view: not just the eugenic elimination of outgroup imperfection and pollution, but enhancement and perfection of the ingroup too. The desire to enhance is the very premise of cognitive genetics, where it is more or less explicit.[5] Explicit too, more often than not, is the 100 per cent fit between individual development and that of the species expressed in socio-economic terms of progress.[6]

Ages means stages: modern developmentalism

Development is both one of the strangest and one of the most commonplace features of the intelligence/disability matrix. What could be more natural to generations schooled in modern biology than the idea that not only the physical organism but the mind, too, evolves and develops – in parallel with the former, by interaction with it, or modelled on it? Evolutionary psychologists do not have to struggle to win a hearing. The full-fledged theory of a mind that develops on an individual basis dates no further back than the mid-nineteenth century, even if its deeper roots lie in Christian notions of salvation.

The ideas of biological evolution *from* and of development *towards* have opposite emphases in relation to time. Biologists these days do not see evolution in terms of developmental goals, but psychologists do use Darwinian 'evolution' to back up the goal-oriented determinism of intellectual 'development'. Darwin himself was diffident about social questions and positively annoyed when people tried to use *On the Origin of Species* to back up theories of progress. Nevertheless, when pushed to discuss the latter, he let the Argument from Design creep back in.[7] This is particularly true of his later *The Descent of Man*. Here, characteristically for an ageing man beset by intellectual fatigue, he reverted to the ideas of the clergyman-biologists he had absorbed at the start of his career, in order to explain social morality (or empathy, as today's paraphrasers call it). Evolutionary psychology, a sub-discipline whose adjective lends spurious hard-science credentials to the questionable ones of the accompanying noun, has no room for such hesitancies. It claims that there is an interaction and/or a parallel between our biological evolution and our evolution from problem-solving to abstract reasoning, and thence to ever-expanding circles of empathy; human groups become integrated through our desire for recognition by our reasoning peers, thereby creating moral norms and adjusting our behaviour to fit.[8]

Darwin also wrote a late essay, 'A Biographical Sketch of an Infant', in which he pictures the development of the child's mind as an ascent out of animality. Yet while Darwin thought the existence of 'idiots' disproved the Argument from Design, he nevertheless expressed little anxiety at all about the fact that he assumed his last and equally loved child, 'born without its full share of intelligence' as he acknowledged, would develop nowhere (the descriptions in his correspondence suggest that Charles Junior had Down's syndrome, though this was a couple of years before Down's creation).[9]

More to the point, developmentalism is famously the brainchild not of the Darwinians but of Piaget. Brainchild in more than a figurative sense: Piaget drew his picture of infancy from the recalled experience of his own upbringing, pasting it solipsistically on the blank page of his general conception of childhood.[10] By now this should come as no surprise. It is simply an extension back into childhood of the standard circularity in discussions of human reason and intelligence, whereby its objective status is belied by the fact that the proposer's own intellect is the model for it. Fond reminiscences of one's own fast-track childhood are common among intelligence enthusiasts.

Piaget famously claimed that mental logic in children develops through distinct and discrete stages. Each is related to their age, and at each ascending level – this time the circularity is a spiral – the subject's intellect displays an ever-greater fit to the objective world around them. Later on he gave his developmental theory of knowledge the grander-sounding name of genetic epistemology. In this oxymoronic phrase the adjective again conveys the flavour of a hard science, the noun a degree of scepticism about what can be known, when Piaget's theory is in fact the reverse: the science is soft, the knowledge claim dogmatic.

Since Piaget is more or less *passé* in psychological and educational circles, let us emphasize again: this book exists to point out the uneradicated roots of various doctrines within the everyday mindset. In inclusion phobia, the idea of development remains a given. Little can be achieved by critical debate about it *within* the human sciences, from some theoretical standpoint or other. Critics have noted that Piaget fails to acknowledge the modular character of intelligence, or that his stages are not watertight.[11] Others note that the material entity of the brain develops too. Standard developmentalism, it is said, relies overmuch on 'crystallized' IQ: it ignores the 'fluidity' of brain matter which starts out, in the young child, as neither localized nor specialized, since it is constantly interfacing with the environment to react back on gene expression as well as on cognition and the 'ultimate cognitive phenotype'.[12] This neuro-constructivist theory of intelligence, using (as so often) disability as its probe, suggests that we employ the term 'development' both for the brain as a material entity and for the intellect. However, this is an abuse of words. By normal development of the brain is meant its *material growth from an initial starting point*, whereas by normal development of cognitive ability is meant the latter's *intellectual progress towards a pre-set goal*. Talk of an 'ultimate' cognitive phenotype is the giveaway, revealing the goal-directed core at the heart of developmentalism.

In short, whatever the criticisms of developmentalism, they leave its tele-ological foundations untouched. Its limitations and contingencies, as we shall see shortly, are historical: its picture of the human individual derives once more from the ladder of nature, albeit following a horizontal axis of time and earthly perfection rather than a vertical one of space and proximity to the divine.

In fact Piaget's contemporary, the Jesuit palaeontologist Pierre Teilhard de Chardin, attempted a fusion between this neo-Darwinian teleology and the older, religious variety. He describes the development of intelligence at species level as the 'humanization' of each individual species member, via 'a continuous series of states ... from the fertilised ovum to the adult'. This marks man's superiority over the other animals, which is an 'ethical necessity' achieved by the 'leap' of intelligent reflection.[13] Man's goal is a divine oneness between the intellect and love. Teilhard's 'series of states' bears similarity to Piaget's notion of a progressive series of age-related developmental stages, each of which must be successfully completed before reaching the next. Piaget too had started out devoutly religious, albeit Protestant (and with Christian socialism in place of love), and his work remains so between the lines. In both Teilhard and Piaget, nature takes over the element of determinism once ascribed to God. Both men saw 'a parallelism between the progress made [by human beings] in the logical and rational organization of knowledge and the corresponding formative psychological processes' of the individual.[14] Piaget maintained that we cannot know the early stages of phylogenic develop-ment – that of the human species in general – because we cannot know the mind of Peking Man (the skull find associated with Teilhard); so let us take advantage instead of the fact that we are surrounded by living beings, young children, whose ontogenic development – that of the individual – is open to observation. This takes us round in another circle, since we are only sur-rounded by living beings of this kind because of our recently acquired belief that children are that subset of human beings who 'develop'.

The catechism had played a key role in Piaget's early religious upbringing and in his transition to a more theoretical outlook.[15] Then, as Binet's teaching assistant, he was introduced to a different kind of assessment in the form of mental age scores.[16] We assume that the testing and assessment of devel-opmental stages comes after the fact, that a prior natural phenomenon (learning disability) exists and someone then comes along and measures it.

Yet historically it is once again the other way round: the idea of developmental stages is a *product* of that administrative and codifying urge which is expressed in the catechism and in the intelligence test alike, themselves phases in the longer-term career of methods of discrimination that preserve ingroup purity. They derive ultimately from that earlier phase of inclusion phobia in which deterministic outgroup categories were religious as well as social, and whose history we shall now examine.

The development of 'development'

When we examine what preceded the appearance of development in the modern human sciences, we come across some familiar-looking terms. For example, medieval theory divided the human intellect (i.e. that particular sector of an all-embracing cosmic intellect which humans could participate in) into two: potential and actual, or active. The familiarity is deceptive. First of all, these were spatial concepts, not temporal ones. The predominant emphasis was vertical. Fallen man needed to rise, not to move onwards (and certainly not towards earthly intellectual perfection, a blasphemous notion in the social context of the time). 'Active' meant, not necessarily an intellect that was busy in the moment, but one that stood in *proximity* to the divine intellect. 'Potential' intellect was not absent albeit imminent; rather, it was present albeit further away.

Moreover, they were quite distinct from each other. Potential intellect referred to ability and active intellect to performance, but ability and performance belonged to strictly separate realms: the latter, as we have already seen, was certainly not the foolproof indicator of the former. Today this has given way to a picture where time predominates, in individual and species development. The child has potential, the perfected adult human has potential *and* actual/active intellect. Hence the category distinction between ability and performance is lost. The childlike adult lacks both. If you cannot perform at the appropriate developmental stage, it means you never had potential in the first place: this absence of potential then helps to construct your extreme outgroup identity.

The fact that the history of the psychology of intelligence reveals no game-changing equivalent to the law of gravity means that there is no sound reason for preferring our modern picture of the mind over the medieval one. It is not a matter of whether one is right and the other wrong. Both are unfalsifiable. Both belong to the realm of myth and gossip out of which inclusion phobia is precipitated. Shamanistic diagnoses of absence/presence are conducted in either period, whether by priestly rite or developmental assessment. What, then, was the concrete historical path from the medieval picture to the modern developmentalist one?

Until the late seventeenth century, the universe, including the human world, was assumed mainly to be static. At that point religion was in the middle of having to cope with a monstrous hangover resulting from a century of over-indulgence in millennialist beliefs. The cure had two ingredients. First, the deadline for the second coming was postponed, so Christians should use the time on earth thus freed up to focus their soul or mind on 'preparation' for the afterlife, rather than cling to the old expectation that grace was conferred by a lightning-bolt that would be occurring any minute now. People began to talk about grace as a quality which individuals could develop for themselves. Second, preparation would not take place (as before) in the will, through simple perseverance; after all, the civil and religious wars of the mid-century had shown that individual wills could cause mayhem. Increasingly, then, preparation was a matter of *reasoning* about one's religion (the expression 'sweet' reason, referring to its calming political effects, dates from this period). This complemented and eventually muscled aside the idea that religion was a matter of revelation. From the mid-nineteenth century onwards the baby went out with the bathwater; reason and intelligence *per se* had won the day, and their paradigmatic occupation was scientific investigation.

Delay and the idea of preparation also opened up the possibility for the numbers of the elect to expand, from a small group to the vast majority of the population. Locke had been reared in a Calvinist environment whose picture of the inner life of human beings was dominated by the deterministic split between the elect and the reprobate we discussed in Chapter 4. In rejecting this picture, he appeared to replace it with that of a universal humanity, when in fact he was *dis*placing the split to somewhere else. The fundamental divide was now between the reasoning majority and a few monstrous exceptions ('changelings', and later, clinically defined idiots). The other main philosophical source of inspiration for modern psychology was Jean-Jacques Rousseau, and a similar shift can be observed in his *Emile, or On Education* and in the French Enlightenment generally, which had absorbed some of the same mentality. Just as the Church of England had its over-enthusiastic predestinarians, so the Catholic church had a wing, known as the Jansenists, who subscribed to a similar doctrine. In opposition to the more inclusive Jesuits who dominated church and state, Jansenism had always been the preference of modernizers. Most of the leading Enlightenment figures had been schooled in some version of it before turning sceptical about religion.

The Jansenists had by then modified their line on election and reprobation. The ensuing watered-down doctrine was a big influence on the young Rousseau. You could now more or less assume that anyone could be saved; Rousseau even denied original sin. Nevertheless there remained the need for some *a priori* exclusion. The Enlightenment philosophers still had in the back of their minds their tutors' attempts to escape the frying-pan of zealous predestinarian divisiveness without toppling into the fire of Jesuit inclusiveness. In predestination-lite we can see the sources of the familiar modern phenomenon of 'inclusion-but': the endorsement of inclusion as a principle only so long as it has a loophole.

One virulent offshoot of the controversies around election involved children. If a child was elect, that status was already fixed before conception. Nevertheless, did it still remain for God to infuse saving grace into them at some point in their earthly lives? If so, when? What were the signs? How could infants dying at birth exhibit faith? These were questions devout parents asked themselves the moment a child was born, in an era when early death was a common event. The residue of deterministic ideas about predestination explains something about *Emile*. His teacher's eureka moment comes when he observes the boy, in one precise activity, reaching and exercising the level of reason that was entirely appropriate to his age.[17] It could not have come earlier and should not come later. Rousseau's idea of development (and following him, Binet's and Piaget's) is at root a response to the question, at what age can we presume election in a child? He writes about Nature's 'gift of education', a conscious transposition from what had previously been God's 'gift of grace'. Nature is a metaphor for the possibility of earthly perfection – social as well as individual – through man's discovery there of his own rationality. Grace, no longer coming instantly from God, now became a developmental aspect of the individual nature. And the position formerly occupied by the reprobate child, the one to whom grace was denied, was now occupied by the child who does not reach the appropriate stage.

This shift also appears in the main eighteenth-century educational authorities such as Isaac Watts in Britain and Jonathan Edwards in the USA. These men's focus was still primarily on the afterlife. They introduced Locke's new picture of human reasoning, which for him had been merely the groundwork for demonstrating humankind's grand religious destiny, into popular literature on schooling, childrearing and behaviour. Their writings outlined the personal qualities all respectable citizens should aspire to develop along the way in readiness for salvation. In France, Binet's mental age scores can be seen as a belated playing out of this. It reveals the tight link between modern notions of a universal humanity (in his case, a universal state schooling) and the exclusions it still necessarily involves. As we have already seen, the existence of exceptions was an absolute presupposition for Binet, regardless of what characterized them. In the cultural legacy he inherited this meant people marked out for damnation in a literal sense. It had been impossible to know for sure who was reprobate and who not, so it was important to look for proxy signs for absence of 'sanctification' in certain people. As we shall see in the next chapter, this function, first fulfilled by the catechism, was transformed organically into developmental assessment and IQ testing.

Development and social history

The idea of development was already inscribed in perceptions of social and religious status and their everyday operations. The practical socio-economic activity and local civic mentality of newly literate populations favoured the rise of development, since a provincial petty bourgeois class was already running local public life and it had aspirations. It had achieved this status as early as the fifteenth and sixteenth centuries, by learning the skills promoted earlier by the clerical caste. At a mundane level, the socio-economic and religious elements were not separate. The Geneva of Calvin's elect was the New York of its day, funding the late sixteenth century's explosion of banking and finance capital. (Rousseau too was born there, and Piaget nearby, who went on to become director of the city's Rousseau Institute.) Some element of learning disability and ability was therefore already embedded in everyday notions of reprobation and election, even if intelligence would take a few generations to become sanctified in its own right and to substitute fully for grace.

The church found ways of accommodating such secular skills within the idea of election through the gift of grace. Guides to godly behaviour increasingly stressed the obligation to have a practical, skilled vocation or 'calling'. Originally there was only a 'general' calling to obey the word of God. This was later supplemented by specific callings that mapped existing social relations: the rich man in his castle, the poor man at his gate, plus an entire system of fixed economic occupations gradually adopting their own hierarchy. By around 1600, it had also spawned the idea of *growth within* one's calling by the exercise of another kind of gift, namely one's personal talents and aptitudes, which usually involved some kind of cleverness. And so it became possible to conceive of a characteristic group of creatures lacking those gifts, and to set them alongside or even with the characteristics of the existing, reprobate outgroup. Even before the idea took hold that faith was not an instantaneous lightning-strike but something one developed by exercising one's reason, the quotidian detail of civic life, urban trade and capitalist expansion had started to offer their own kind of regeneration, justification and sanctification, and of developmental aspirations. Personal, religious and social all at once, these marked the onset of the modern era's own specific norms of upward social mobility.

Out of these pragmatic roots the idea of the calling, and of a category of persons incapable of a calling, became central to theories of society and religion. One of the period's key works in this respect, translated into English and widely read across Europe in the late sixteenth century, was Juan Huarte's *The Examination of Men's Wits.*[18] Although historians have exaggerated the book's modern resonances, it does contain a primitive developmentalist account of education and apprenticeship. Meanwhile Huarte's contemporary William Perkins, one of Calvinist Europe's leading theologians, a thorough dogmatist about election and reprobation and thus about one's destiny in the afterlife, himself brought earthly callings into this context. An apprentice's place in socio-economic life should be regarded not simply as a matter of his personal fate but as a result of his being the 'fittest' and most 'able' to do the job. This demanded assessment ('trial of gifts') and meritocratic advancement ('free election without particularity'). Human beings are individually responsible not only for their relationship to God and the next life (the classic Protestant theory) but also for developing the abilities that will enable them to make their way through this life – this too is part of renewing their souls.[19] They are thus responsible for social reform in the here and now. Earthly as well as heavenly gifts can improve a static, sinful social order.

This applied to children too. 'Even in his first years' a child 'does affect some one particular calling', says Perkins. Religious tracts and self-help behavioural manuals of the time used the animal- and plant-breeding metaphors that

Galton would one day pick up on, recommending the improvement and development of human stock. Elite pontificating about honour and election was matched by practical advice from people like the Lowestoft fish traders who warned their fellow-citizens that 'no greater profit [can] arise to the commonwealth than the instruction of youth ... truly that commonwealth is miserable, wherein the tillage of infancy is neglected'.[20] Development into adulthood through apprenticeship was a yielding of interest on capital invested for the future; the richer a trawlerman got, the more it blotted out the contaminating odour of mackerel, especially on his children. The sanctity of social and religious status trappings, of airs and graces, could then be transferred to the mundane cleverness involved in parochial, petty bourgeois advancement and upward mobility. The idea of perfection, once located in the past, in the glorious aristocratic ancestor or in Adam before the Fall, was reassigned to the developmental future.

This solved tensions over the rapid inflation of titles and honours that went with the rise of the merchant class who purchased them. Their own families were usually only a generation away from belonging to the idiot outgroup. People just clambering on to the first rung of the gentry ladder claimed to possess 'virtue', a suitably catch-all term that dominated discussions of human behaviour from the sixteenth to eighteenth centuries. Hinting at the military virtue of fake aristocratic ancestors might not be enough to ensure ingroup membership, so it had to be supplemented by acquiring the humanist virtue of 'learning'. Preserving ancestral glory became less important than investing in a staged future growth. Intellectual perfectibility, from being the quality of a rapidly expanding elite, would by the end of the eighteenth century become that of the whole species. Thus was born the idea of a progressive universal history. Universal it may be, but the species in that sense still has to remove its last vestiges of anxiety by purging itself of an outgroup, however small, whose individual inability to develop is now represented as the greatest hindrance to the social development of everyone else.

Notes

1 J. Clapton (2009). *A Transformatory Ethic of Inclusion*. Rotterdam: Sense.
2 J. Pring (2014). 'Inclusion is only right for some disabled children, says EHRC', *Disability News Service*, 24.
3 E. Young-Bruehl (2012). *Childism: Confronting Prejudice against Children*. New Haven, CT: Yale University Press.
4 P. Alderson (2013). *Childhoods Real and Imagined*. Abingdon: Routledge; P. Aries (1962). *Centuries of Childhood*. New York: Vintage.
5 See for example R. Nisbett et al. (2012). 'Intelligence: new findings and theoretical developments', *American Psychologist* 67(2), 130–160; C. Shulman and N. Bostrom (2014). 'Embryo selection for cognitive enhancement: curiosity or game-changer?' *Global Policy* 5(1), 85–92.
6 See for example A. Sandberg and J. Savulescu (2011). 'The social and economic impacts of cognitive enhancement', in J. Savulescu et al. (eds), *Enhancing Human Capacities*. New York: Wiley.

7 R. Young (1985). *Darwin's Metaphor*. Cambridge: Cambridge University Press.
8 See for example T. Suddendorf (2014). *The Gap: The Science of What Separates Us from Other Animals*. New York: Basic Books.
9 Cited in A. Desmond and J. Moore (1991). *Darwin*. London: Michael Joseph, p. 446.
10 B. Bradley (1989). *Visions of Infancy: Critical Introduction to Child Psychology*. Cambridge: Polity.
11 Howard Gardner (2008). 'Wrestling with Jean Piaget, my paragon'. *The World Question Center*, www.edge.org/q2011/q11_index.html. Retrieved 11 September 2014.
12 A. Karmiloff-Smith (2006). 'The tortuous route from genes to behaviour: a neuro-constructivist approach', *Cognitive, Affective, and Behavioral Neuroscience* 6(1), 9–17.
13 P. Teilhard de Chardin (1959). *The Phenomenon of Man*. London: Harper, pp. 164ff.
14 J. Piaget (1968). *Genetic Epistemology*. New York: Columbia University Press.
15 See F. Vidal (1994). *Piaget before Piaget*. Cambridge, MA: Harvard University Press.
16 F. Wesley (1989). 'Developmental cognition before Piaget: Alfred Binet's pioneering experiments', *Developmental Review* 9, 58–63.
17 J.-J. Rousseau (1762/1979). *Emile, or On Education*. New York: Basic Books.
18 J. Huarte (1594/1969). *The Examination of Men's Wits*. Amsterdam: Da Capo Press.
19 Cited in Withington, *The Politics of Commonwealth*, p. 114.
20 Cited in Withington, p. 115.

7   Assessment

Within the UK's education system, which segregates children from adults, is Verdant Meadows, a segregated special school for children with severe learning difficulties. Within segregated Verdant Meadows is a further segregated special unit for those with challenging behaviour. I can see a large wall chart. In the vertical column are the students' names, in the horizontal the weeks of the term. In the boxes are numbers indicating points scored for good behaviour (from what I observe, this means any behaviour that is passive or does not challenge the system). Names of class members are ranked not alphabetically but in order of points scored. To make it look more specialist, the points have been organized around a mean score. At the top is Rafael, whose score every week is around 120. At the bottom is Andrew, whose score barely ever reaches double figures. Andrew, already ejected from one situation, needs to bear in mind that there is probably no special school or institution, or special unit within it, that itself does not patrol its own boundaries and eject accordingly. Like the model village within the model village, a segregated institution can only replicate within itself the symptoms, such as an obsession with number, that are present in the initial general disorder.

Carl Nightingale has written about the universality of 'city-splitting' in general, and about the direct line that can be traced from ancient temple compounds to modern forms of geographical and social cleansing. 'Surely this cannot have been a precedent for any conceivable form of modern segregation?' asked one sceptical reviewer of this book.[1] Yes it can. Inasmuch as it is the methodologies of assessment that are cross-historical rather than the concept of intellectual disability as such, these can be located in the planning of physical spaces too, and in what Gabel calls the 'morbid geometrism' that accompanies morbid rationalism. It is in those methodologies, rather than in the content of labels, that grand historical schemes will work.

Yet the individual's position outside the closed circle of an ordinary institution reflects their position outside a conceptual circle too, and such circles have in the past been fuzzy. The idea of a ladder of nature was once just that: an idea. It was a universal given. Therefore it needed no pseudo-scientific verification. Nor did your personal ingroup position on it. True, law and administration before the modern era were sharply discriminatory; they could forbid you to sit in the front pews at church or wear clothes that were above your estate.

But they did not produce outgroups in the 'extreme' sense that aligns status boundaries with those of the species, nor purely on the invisible, intangible basis of how something called the mind did or did not operate.

We have already seen that through to the end of the seventeenth century individual anomalies thrown up by biological nature were still seen as 'accidents', and that the boundaries of natural categories were soft-edged; this still held true even when people outside the social elite were being described as animal-like. The reason for this was that there existed a second classificatory system which their apparent bestiality did not contradict. This was the much harder-edged criterion of *essences*. It chimed with the biblical idea of the human species as a 'lump' rather than an aggregate of individuals. 'Essence' guaranteed the species membership of all individuals *prima facie*. Even the growing bureaucratic mentality of the early modern era did not exhibit the virulence of the phobia that the last century and a half has exhibited. What is so different about our own world is how desperately and uniformly an extreme outgroup matters. The desperation displays itself in the use of statistically based assessment as the tool for exclusion. In this obsessive compulsion, madness has finally become the method. In a further, typical delusion, a reciprocal relationship between two sets of people whose separate identities are in any case merely notional becomes skewed into a relationship between an ingroup that defines itself as observer and an outgroup defined by its being observed. Its members resemble the sinners in the lowest circle of Dante's hell, whose loss of humanity is represented by being frozen into the ice as helpless specimens for dispassionate observation by passing travellers on the road to perfection of the intellect in paradise.

One of the absolute presuppositions we have noted is that *ability* can only be inferred from an observable, external realm of measurable *performance*. The two are collapsed into each other, eliding the category distinction between them that was routine among classical and Renaissance thinkers. Like present-day critics such as Martha Nussbaum, they saw ability as constituting membership of society or a social group, not as an external and measurable contribution to it.[2] The reduction of assessment to measurement puts the final scientific veneer on inclusion phobia. Yet even in physics or chemistry measurement is always an 'emergent property', not something that can be used in circular fashion to verify whatever one wants to verify.[3] And if so, how much the more so with things like intelligence and learning disability that have no stable subject-matter, and over several generations can shed most of their skin? Assessment is instrumental and nothing else: uninterested in whether or not what it is observing is something with a real existence in nature, and whether or not that thing is always in a process of transformation into something else.

Morbid rationalism and cognitive ability testing

Like Piaget's developmentalism, IQ has been largely debunked outside of cognitive genetics, at the same time as penetrating ever more deeply into the everyday mindset. Yesterday's theory is today's rather more powerful knee-jerk. Thus it is the thing that impacts on people's lives – as in court rulings such as 'the victim/defendant has a mental age of x'. The quarrels about IQ and cognitive ability testing have been plentiful and noisy. Critics claim them to be culturally biased against black people, women, or working-class children; the characteristics of intelligence are dynamic, not fixed or thus measurable; tests can only measure what the tester decides is important, not any supposedly general intelligence; tests ought to measure a, b and c rather than x, y and z; test results are not historically constant; we value what we can measure when we should be measuring what we value. In practice, all these criticisms imply a request from the learning-disabled outgroup: please let us in. Polite requests do not work with the insane; the very act of requesting validates the excluder's outlook on the world. The criticisms may be true, but they skate over the essential point, which is that cognitive ability tests are needed only because an ingroup/outgroup boundary like learning disability is needed; they do not feature in inclusive environments, as there is no point in their being there. Tests are essential to any society suffering from inclusion phobia inasmuch as they are bureaucratic details which on the one hand are pointless (the people they are used on are already labelled and suspect) yet on the other are needed because they display the 'rituals of order' typical of totalitarian regimes.[4] Despite their redundancy, they act as reassurances in a disordered situation.

It is true that IQ testing, at least in the UK, is less and less used by educational psychologists (and even DSM makes a point of marking levels of severity by adaptive functioning rather than IQ). Its segregating function in special education has nevertheless been replaced by decision-making from the headteacher, who is now the one to make the call as to whether something is moderate, severe or profound. Even figleaf science is no longer seen to be necessary, in a system so accepting of arbitrary administrative writ. Moreover, as IQ exits educational psychology it enters cognitive genetics, whose aims are eugenic. Eliminating the reproduction of undesirables – the original impulse behind sterilization and segregated schooling – has been pushed back for practical purposes to the pre-natal stage. In short, IQ is not old hat. It is entirely fit for purpose: that is, the irrational purpose of the dominant ideology for which it was designed, and to whose segregated structures it is intrinsic because it is related to a particular definition of what human beings are. This explains why every successful demolition of its conceptual basis in questions of race and gender continues to be followed by a revival. It is not a new hat that is required but a new head, cured of the phobia.

As ritual, in an anthropological sense, assessment incorporates shamanism and magic. Rituals screen for contamination. Fom catechisms and systems of heraldic symbols through to the bell curve, the driver is the *bottom* end of the ladder. Ascent of a numerical scale proceeds in parallel with ascent of a natural, hierarchical one, consisting of relative distance from the feared animality of the impostors below. We have already seen that the seventeenth-century concept of a natural disability of the intellect preceded and was the very precondition for that of a natural intellectual ability. The same then applies to the methods for verifying it. Assessment in action is unidirectional: it only proceeds upwards, that is, to the point where it proves that someone *can't* do something.

Testing came into being not in order to measure intelligence as such, anywhere along the scale, but precisely in order to quarantine. Anyone who has sat with someone with learning difficulties, usually a young person or child, as they are being taken through a test will know that the tester is not finding out what they can do, even within the crabbed space of what a test considers the most important aspect of being human. Like the shaman, the tester is looking for the point of *absence*. This point forms a boundary, a conceptual segregation aligned with practical, social segregation and the removal of certain people from the pure intelligent space that is the ingroup. It is usually dressed up as help for the outgroup member rather than decontamination of the ingroup, and is how historians have presented Binet's invention of the mental age score. It begs the question why, if help and support are needed, they have to take place in segregated settings.

Morbid rationalism, the obsession with number, was described by Minkowski as typical of schizoid states, and by Gabel as typical of ideological standpoints in general, especially of those that are in power. It is part of how they avoid contemplating their own eventual fall from grace or any refutation of their supposed rationality, by ignoring history. The sense of change over time is marginalized, thus omitting a view of the whole. What Gabel calls the 'spatialization of time' favours unwarranted mathematical extrapolations that rigidify the present moment into a static system. How can it change if it is already perfect? This is characteristic not only of disordered individuals but also of political and especially utopian thought.

Morbid rationalism in action

What does morbid rationalism look like in action? Gabel describes it in one of his psychiatric patients.[5] While it is one man's own individual mental illness, it also reflects his absorption of certain recognizably modern, totalitarian features of social organization. He has issued laws for an imaginary state, while remaining totally mute about his past. He wears 'papal insignia' with nine stars on his sleeve, and heads up a theocratic system with the utilitarian purpose of creating universal happiness. 'There are five Popes. I am first.' Who is the second Pope?

> They go from sixteen to sixteen ... One is fifty-five years old, the next seventy-one, the next eighty-seven, and so it goes. When one dies, there is another from sixteen. It follows. If the one who is eighty-seven does not die, that makes six popes ... The popes are the five leaders of France ... There are five cardinals per continent, which makes twenty-five cardinals. There are five archbishops in each archbishopric, five bishops in each bishopric. In each bishopric there are four deputy bishops. In each sub-bishopric there are five archdeacons, which makes twenty archdeacons,

as heads of each local authority. Each local authority has four parishes with five priests in each parish, as parish chiefs. I'm the one who set this system up, for the purposes of more energetic government.

Crucially, the state cannot promote happiness as long as it contains 'heretics': specifically, for this patient, 'krauts', 'anarchists' and 'protestants' – they all amount to the same thing – who must be ejected in order for the system to work.

Any system of controlling and hence judging human beings will always makes perfect sense as long as it meets two conditions. First, that everyone accepts its premise as rational. Second, that the system does not contain that which has already defined it as a system, i.e. the outgroup. Thus proof against pollution, it is then free to follow a rational detailed pattern based on numerical hierarchy.

Gabel's pseudo-Pope resembles devisers of other utopian schemes. Take for example the author of a 1916 outline for a world assembly. His questionably rational premise was that the more intelligent an ethnic group is, the more votes it should have; some should have none at all. The constitution of his utopian state extended eugenic and developmentalist principles to those of social organization: 'The desire for a sound and honest World Government by all mankind and earnest effort for biological race-betterment by each of the several nations are two movements which would interact powerfully to strengthen each other.' People 'from generation to generation … must improve their own hereditary equipment'. World government could therefore only work through sterilization of the unintelligent. Moreover, his system of six continental subdivisions for world government required its administrative centre to be located in exactly the right place, where intelligence was at its most advanced. Using statistically mapped criteria, the author worked out that the world capital should lie near the confluence of the Mississippi and Missouri rivers. With due respect to the present-day citizens of Kirksville Mo., this was not an obvious choice. But it was the author's own birthplace and where he lived and worked. Moreover, he was no asylum patient. He was Dr Harry Laughlin, principal scientific adviser to the House of Representatives committee on immigration, director of the USA's leading eugenics laboratory between the two world wars, and writer of the draft sterilization law which, enacted by numerous American states, would go on to provide the chief inspiration for Rüdin's Law on the Prevention of Hereditarily Diseased Offspring.[6]

The ideal human being at the centre of the childless and epileptic Laughlin's world state, with its pursuit of happiness through hereditary enhancement of intelligence, was himself, just as it was for Gabel's patient. In the formulation first set down by Locke, madness consists in correct reasoning from false premises; hence in Gogol's *Diary of a Madman*, once a downtrodden pen-pusher realizes he is King of Spain everything else that previously puzzled him about the world suddenly becomes crystal clear. Rational or not, what we can say about the premises in all these cases is that they are similar. All three forms of status – papal, intelligent and monarchical – share the fact that they are all personal representations of the divinity on earth.

It is true that we now claim to have recovered from certain symptoms of Laughlin's disorder. His view of intelligence as colour-coded – his world voting system meant that 'one man in the USA is equal to more than 25 times the representation value of one man in India' – is now deemed unscientific by many, though it remains alive in the psychometric community, extending well beyond the obsessive tail-pulling of the self-styled 'hereditarian' (racist) psychologists such as J. Philippe Rushton. Either way, psychometrically oriented psychologists will endorse, even 'with reluctance', the idea that black people or women have lower IQs and are therefore biochemically different, on the grounds that respect for the evidence demands it, although they reject accusations of prejudice because the evidence is based on averages and therefore does not say anything about the intelligence of a black or female individual.[7]

Any counter-argument entering the debate about prejudice at this level, and not at the ontological level of intellectual disability itself, is already fatally disarmed. Even for Laughlin and his American contemporaries, race was merely the proxy for a deeper-lying phobia. All that number-crunching about race makes perfect sense as long as the rationality of the hidden premise is accepted: namely, Laughlin's principle of 'inherent intelligence', which *per se* is 'the basis of democracy'. Substitute meritocracy and its exclusions for democracy here, and we have a fair description of the mainstream of current political thought. Once the concepts of intelligence and learning disability are accepted as sound premises, the system can justify any consequent insanities by being couched in terms of number.

Statistical measurement lends an air of objectivity and neutrality. The more perfectly it fits the thing it describes, intelligence, the more that is because of the thing's arbitrary character. The function of number is to represent intellectual ability as the stable premise it is not. That explains why, as we saw earlier, experimental psychologists can be dismissive about the need to define intelligence, since definition lies in the sphere of measurement alone: not even because number itself is an exact realm, but rather because there is simply nowhere else for a definition of intelligence to lie. In the early twentieth century Karl Pearson, who contributed more than anyone to raising the assessment of intelligence to a statistical level, went further. He claimed that correlation reigns supreme so far as to render irrelevant all discussion of things correlated and why they might be as they are – thus rendering irrelevant too the very rationality of the premise. In our understanding of intelligence, any applied system of numbers that makes arithmetical sense is entirely rational just as long as we do not question the reality of what it is the system illustrates – and the final triumph of inclusion phobia's pathology arrives with the explicit acknowledgement of this by those suffering from it.

Exclusion belongs to the 'language game' of number, as Wittgenstein would have termed it.[8] In this game, the claims of experimental psychology with no family resemblance to exact sciences such as biology and medicine are fed into the ears of government, which borrows the practice of randomized control trials from physiological medicine (where variables can be eliminated) and applies them to social policy and the school classroom (where they cannot).[9] As we already saw with family research, the possibilities for non-quantitative research are siphoned off by restyling a bit of quantitative research 'qualitative': for example, in quality of life indicators, whose usefulness and very validity lie in the fact that they can be counted. Assessment for intelligence is an illicit borrowing from the medical model of assessment for disease. In biological science measurement is one thing, classification another. Ordering systems do not exclude. They are taxonomic. That is, they classify species at a horizontal, value-neutral level. Biologists, at least those not manipulated by the cognitive world view, complain about the skewing of research funds towards genetics precisely on the grounds that it tells us only why things go wrong instead of why they differ.[10] The very insertion of a component called mind switches that ordering system from the horizontal to the vertical. A value hierarchy appears, already fully formed inasmuch as it is dredged from a mindset imbued with the medieval ladder of nature. Any values are *a priori*. There is no numerical assessment without a pre-existing assumption of hierarchy.

Number and its aura of science clothe the phobia in a pure rhetoric about status; the act of assessment is the rational justification of an irrational premise. Of course the word assessment covers many different aspects of the mind sciences. There are certain individual abilities that may well be judged, on an epistemologically or ethically sound basis, as greater or lesser. In assessments of intelligence, however, the circularity of the schizoid conceptual process is clear. Like the ancient symbol of the crocodile eating its own tail, a disability assessment does not just come after the disability, it also came before: it assesses something that is a product of itself. This is not even a feedback loop, since assessment feeds nothing back into the circle, even to reinforce it and certainly not to correct it. It is more like what the computing world calls a recursion; that is to say, the learning disability identified within each individual arises and is endlessly repeated within the general definition to which it belongs. Hence, in practical terms, assessments become obsessive-compulsive automata; the same words are cut-and-pasted into educational and care assessments from one actual individual to the next, thus showing assessment to be an entirely quantitative process. Individual persons fit the system they are required to fit.

Morbid rationalism also exhibits itself in the inverse correlation between the size of the extreme outgroup and the threat this poses, where the more its numbers tend to zero, the greater the threat. This is an obviously paranoid symptom: in social terms, a moral panic. It is not only an unwarranted extrapolation, it also spawns a contradiction: the smaller the actual number, the greater the potential number. An argument against inclusive schooling that recurs incessantly in local policy discussions is the warning that there are big increases of *them* coming through the system, needing to be dealt with. The specific characteristics of *them*, in the upcoming age-group, will tend to correspond with whatever moral panic is going around at the time (at the moment, autism and attention deficit). The schizoid contradiction here is easy enough to spot, but only once one has opted out of the moral panic and morbid rationalism that dominate the field.

Morbid rationalism and rebellion

The geometrical figure of a circle is defined by what lies outside the line: its area is bound or limited. This applies to the geography of institutions as well as psychological objects. You have an assessment to be put in a different *place*. Assessment leads to 'different', 'other', 'specialist' and eventually to separated, segregated and eliminated, even though the same energy (or less) could be used to find out who people are, what their aspirations are, and to plan for them to stay inside the circle where they may contribute as much as anyone else. Socially determined and historically contingent people's position outside of a conceptual and institutional circle may be, but since the individuals concerned are precisely those deemed incapable of conceptualizing anything, where would any challenge come from? Who is there to express a sane, non-ideological perspective?

Assessment is a successful defensive manoeuvre, a fortified circular emplacement behind which the vast numbers of the ingroup protect themselves from being contaminated by the few. It is necessary because the outgroup itself, by its very existence, might reveal that the idea of intelligence is an attribution of value and nothing else. Above all, a critical perspective from beyond the circle might reveal the disjuncture between being a member of an ingroup and being a member of a natural species.

In fact this discussion remains theoretical. In practice, an objective view from beyond the circle is possible. As we have seen, history gives us one such view. However, the present moment too affords such a view. People with learning difficulties themselves, and those close to them, can articulate it. Observing the assessment of 12-year-old Bradley, who has Down's syndrome, I watch the educational psychologist put pencil and paper in front of him and ask him to draw something (by which she means anything). Bradley throws the pencil down and folds his arms. His reaction makes it clear to me that this very laid-back young man is used to having to deal with such behaviour. He remains silent to the end, and the psychologist finishes with a test on his logical grasp of 'same' and 'different', that staple of the assessment diet. Her final question is 'What's the difference between these two toys, Bradley? Is this the same as that one, or is it different?' He stays silent, but as he leaves the room with his mother he turns and asks, scowling: 'What's the difference between a person and a brick?'

Bradley has stood his assessor's reification of him on its head and turned it back against her. Despite an ability/performance score of zero, he was able to perceive the static and clinically disordered nature of the ingroup's thought-processes, and that is because he was perfectly positioned to do so. This takes us back to Piaget. It is well-known that in administering a test, a relationship is formed with the person being tested. The relationship with Bradley was clearly dysfunctional, but the dysfunction can operate in pleasanter ways. When Piaget repeated questions of children, they 'seemed to want to please him by providing different answers'.[11] Despite the fact that these were ethical responses, aimed helpfully (unlike Bradley's) at accommodating and perhaps ameliorating the autistic immobility of Piaget's own personality and its morbid rationalism, Piaget presented their inconsistencies as evidence of developmental immaturity.

Assessment in history: the beginnings

Intelligence and its disabilities become real categories partly *because* they are measurable. Without modern learning disability, no testing – but also: without testing, no learning disability. Alongside discontinuity in the target categories of inclusion phobia there is its own continuity exhibited in the methodologies of discrimination. To see assessment for what it is, we need to set it in the broader context of the increasingly tightened codifications of extreme outgroup status, of whatever content, from the late medieval period and still more sharply from 1500 onwards – after which assessment takes on a life of its own. The historical constant is the building of a rational system on an irrational premise and the use of a numerical or symbolic language to close off the circle, even as the outgroups it creates are changing. Just as the idea of a specifically human intelligence, being the new status claim, emerged dialectically out of an interaction and competition between the earlier ones of social and religious status, so too its assessment methods emerged seamlessly, albeit in clearly discernible phases, from the forms of assessment used to measure honour and grace.

The ingroup of the modern era, the intellectually able, has absorbed in its attitude to its extreme outgroup the self-referring status anxieties that once belonged to far smaller elites. In the sixteenth century, the majority of ordinary adults did not themselves worry about whether they were elect or not. Only the social and religious hierarchy had such a high and mighty but consequently anxiety-ridden view of the basic principles of status. Later, during the English civil wars and revolution, a desire to be among the elect did seize groups of laypeople and commoners, but even then, most of the population did not let it go to their heads. Nor did the fishmongers and greengrocers who in the absence of 'blood' gentry held power in the provincial cities go so far as to think themselves blood descendants of Hector of Troy, as the duelling wing of the metropolitan gentry did, or of King Solomon, as its intellectual wing did (Robert Boyle and Isaac Newton both thought this).

Honourable, titled families were subjected to regular visitations by a commission of heraldic experts. It practised on this small sector of the population a primitive form of statistics ('state numbers') collected for the fiscal and private purposes of the Tudor exchequer. As with IQ, the *measurability* of honour constituted the *proof* of its reality. It had its own specific science to do the measuring, called Blazon.[12] This was 'the most refined part of natural philosophy', the latter being what we now call the exact sciences. It was exact as geometry. It ranked you and your family's place in the social order by a hierarchy of heraldic symbols, publicly displayed as coats of arms. This was what justified passing your title to your children. Your entitlement to a coat was recorded for legal purposes on pro formas containing pictorial symbols above and itemizing the family tree below. Number was involved in the 'quartering' of symbols, the multiples of ancestral generations and their own coats of arms.

Heraldry, though it sounds and was deliberately engineered to sound as if it denoted ancient ancestry, was in fact one of the first forms of modern population control to supersede ramshackle feudal ones. With it came the official registration of marriages, initially among the elite. While it designated status rather than actual property, the two had equal importance. The gentleman or gentlewoman, or their fathers, selected a partner whose social status and biological inheritance (blood) could be verified by Blazon, just as the middle-class single mother selects the sperm of someone whose high intelligence can be verified by an IQ score. The core purpose of the Commission of Heralds, however, was not to confer honours but to detect impostors. Not only would they pollute the ingroup, their presence threatened to expose the fact that even supposedly authentic families' historical origins were often as common as muck ('newly arisen from the dunghill' was the phrase used at the time). Most could not trace their genteel origins back more than two or three generations.

In religion, the aim of catechism was similarly to weed out pollutant reprobates. Their identifying mark was hypocrisy, which in the religious terms of the time meant to be good at faking piety. The edification of the elect – which featured in the catechism – was no doubt an aim, but it could not be achieved without the elimination of contaminant elements. (Galton's theory of avoiding regression to the mean in order to enhance the white races would eventually spring from this mentality.) Reprobation, like social vulgarity and like learning disability, was the prior category, out of which elect, ingroup status was precipitated; theologically speaking, the elect were merely reprobates who had been pardoned. Grace was as real as honour, and proof of this, once again, was again that it could be measured in the human individual. The elect were a determinate number that could not go up or down. It was sometimes claimed, moreover, that the amount of grace each person possesses was quantifiable. Elect individuals could therefore be ranked on a hierarchical scale with a systematic queue at the pearly gates and an 'order of the just' numbered from 1 downwards.

Assessment in education

Assessment and development are integral to each other. The morbid rationalism of quantification was at root a system of ejection that over time found its way into university and school exam systems. The catechism, the assessment-based instrument of sanctification (i.e. of checking that a person, once elect, had not lapsed), became part of the testing regime in education. The general curriculum including literacy and numeracy, was taught through it.

A ubiquitous school textbook, *The ABC with Catechism*, was in use from the mid-sixteenth century till the late mid-eighteenth – following which, the word catechism acquired the secondary meaning of a crammer or set of revision notes.[13]

The first school inspectors were the local clergy, called in to hear teachers test children on their catechism and what they were learning through it. The schoolroom of the Southwell workhouse in 1824, for example, records a blackboard in which the letters of the alphabet and the numbers 1–10 are set out at the top, and underneath are the words of a hymn:

> Happy the child whose tender years
> Receive instruction well,
> Who hates the sinner's paths and fears
> The road that leads to hell.

When, in the latter part of the century, the first formal psychologists began to be interested in children, their starting point was not the principles of an as yet non-existent subdiscipline, educational psychology; rather, they began by observing the existing assessment methods of class teachers and then absorbed them within the new discipline.[14] Mental age scores and IQ are thus an organic refinement of the church catechism. Both are alert to the possibility that some children might be hellbound. Damnation can be intellectual as well as moral. Fakes are weeded out for segregation. The whole point behind the invention of the moron category at the end of the nineteenth century was that morons operated with enough intellectual ability to fool you into thinking they were normal. Assessment underwrites category boundaries among children with statistical evidence, and this then feeds into presuppositions of a more general kind about an intellectual hierarchy within the ingroup. The Calvinist church has now been succeeded at the head of the queue of the elect by the Russell Group and the Ivy League. Blazon has been replaced by exam grades. Pseudo-scientific methods of discrimination have given way to the chi-squared truths of IQ.

Scholastic assessment is also important because the discipline of clinical psychology as a whole has roots in special education. Though it was partly also an extension of 'abnormal psychology', the American psychologist Lightner Witmer, usually credited with founding it or at least of coining the phrase and to some extent thus inventing the discipline, had started out in special education; his work only became 'clinical' inasmuch as he did not observe supposedly difficult children in an educational context of any kind. They came to him instead, out of that environment, and into a specialist one that eventually drew in adults too.

Assessment as sanctification

Given a degree of continuity in inclusion phobia's assessment methods, we can track shifts in the nature of successive extreme outgroups by seeing what those methods alight on each time. Obsessive compulsion with number in the study of human beings was one of the key movers in bringing learning disability to the centre ground. To see how this came about, we can look at another of its precursor concepts, this time taken from medicine. Although doctors were latecomers in the field, by the nineteenth century they would be swamping it.

In medicine, the centre ground had long been occupied by melancholy. From the middle ages onwards, it had been the paradigmatic mental disorder, transcending both madness and any budding elements of learning disability. It was a flexible term with many different, shifting meanings. Originally a bodily condition (excess of 'black bile') and capable of being manic as well as depressive, it eventually became an intellectual and emotional disorder focused on the latter, identified by sloth – at a time when the burgeoning concept of human intelligence was increasingly being identified with speed of reaction and thought. By the later seventeenth century melancholy was also coming to overlap religious and social categories, being used to describe transgressive behaviour patterns such as atheism, political dissent, or religious despair.

In these latter senses, melancholy was seen by some as a collective characteristic of social groups – of women, for example. Being a melancholic was unlike being a reprobate, as it was not deterministic; rather, it belonged to the soft-edged concept of human nature, a kind of second nature with grey areas that *might* be curable if people could only knuckle down to self-improvement. Nevertheless, in the minds of pastors and teachers it tended to coalesce with reprobation and thus determinism. The transformation of melancholy along with reprobation into the new, pathological idiocy, involved a numerical system that would feed into the beginnings of cognitive assessment. That system was double-entry bookkeeping.

This was already inherent in the idea of the calling. When early Protestant businessmen and bankers kept accounts, they represented this activity to themselves as recording their contribution to God's purposes on earth. Melancholy resulted in failure to contribute, and likewise lent itself to counting. Its 'atheistic' element consisted of despair about the possibility of one's personal receipt of grace, which might end in doubt about the possibility that there was a God. People had begun to *count the signs* of grace in themselves; here are the historical roots of all those guides to knowing your own IQ or how far along the autism spectrum you are. And increasing anxiety about one's own status ('Am I saved?') led from the rough-and-ready assessment of the catechism to a numerical method. If the catechism partly existed to ascertain whether people were still sanctified and had not lapsed, after the decline in millennialist beliefs the term came to denote more concrete rewards and sufferings on this earth. Clarissa Harlowe, in Samuel Richardson's famous novel, constantly writes about her afflictions being 'sanctified' for her rather than causes for despair, meaning she could credit them to the incomings side of the double entry page and her down payment on a place in heaven.

Protestant notions of the examined self had always had a role for learning. While to begin with the word indicated something objective, a body of unchangeable biblical text, it was gradually complemented by learning as a subjective process within the individual. People began to count as signs of ingroup membership the *number of hours* they spent in 'meditations', i.e. in examining their inner status. They advanced their learning by probing the possibility that they were elect. In fact one of the chief origins of the turn towards epistemology in modern Western thought generally lies in this doubt about one's elect status. The very word *psychologia*, first coined in the 1580s to defend the doctrine of the soul's immortality, also promoted a new interest in individual self-knowledge. This accompanied the anxious search for decontaminated signs of grace in oneself, also provoking interest in the precise workings of the minds of others (you wanted to know if your neighbour was saved or damned) and thereby to the very stuff of psychological inquiry.

A continuous path thus leads from past to present, from the assessment of utterly strange things such as honour, grace and medieval melancholy to our utterly taken-for-granted modern ones such as intelligence and learning disability, which will of course one day become strange to our descendants. Originally sanctification – sustainability on the path to salvation – had been as mysterious as election itself; it was a process known only to God. Earthly achievements and understanding, let alone having a tally system for them, had been irrelevant at best and a dangerous diversion at worst. Now, active learning became itself a form of sanctification that you could 'credit' to yourself when totting up an assessable list of reasons why you had a right to live forever. Coinciding with this came a shift in the way logical reasoning was perceived. This too involved counting. The classic medieval unit of human reasoning had been the syllogism, consisting of two premises and a conclusion; there was just one move, towards the conclusion, otherwise it was a static structure. In the seventeenth century the syllogism was replaced by the idea of reasoning as a continuing succession of units, called 'trains of thought' (Hobbes) or 'trains of ideas' (Locke). Trains are temporal sequences that act on each other like billiard balls; they are not structures but *events* in the life of the mind, and therefore more susceptible to counting.

All these changes of method for assessing the internal characteristics of the ingroup involved the reconstruction of the outgroup, and vice-versa. Their function was absorbed in the education system. Mathematics started to replace language as the core skill, even in religious terms, because it consisted in sequences that modelled trains of ideas and helped the student to stay focused.[15] When the syllogism had prevailed, the pathology of excess mobility lay in constantly shifting opinions. Now it lay in constantly wavering attention. Meanwhile, the *exercise* of grace, as Jonathan Edwards called it – no longer a bolt from the blue but an internal self-activation and self-development – consisted in recorded hours of concentrated effort, correlated with likelihood of success. As always, the anxiety was gendered and classed. Both women and labourers in general were particularly prone to melancholy, but were also warned against *too many* hours of mental exercise, which would have been inappropriate to their callings and to their very nature, which was subordinate.

Assessment by catechism was both an external restraint and, complementing this, a stimulus to self-reflection. But even those nonconformist pioneers who sought to make it a model for behavioural control across the population, acknowledged that it had its limits. At first, the subject sought the source of his own value by himself and in himself. But self-reflection could only be validated on the basis of judgment by others. It became a conversation not just with one's personal God but also with like-minded people. Hence the rise of the eighteenth-century epistolary novel, where friends write letters exposing their innermost thoughts and inviting each other to check on their character and motives. Like Clarissa, one audited one's inner self by presenting the mind's accounts for inspection by others. At the same time, the predominance of familial and friendship networks was yielding to a broader civic and public sphere that would now see human beings as a network of commodified equals, and systems of qualitative social reciprocity would be replaced by quantified forms of it within a very large ingroup indeed.

Assessment as the new science of segregation

The relationship between intelligence and learning disability is thus one of the sub-systems of those modern, commodified types of social reciprocity that was formalized with the arrival of psychology as a discipline. In the field of intelligence, the primary application of the principle of equal exchange came with the normal curve of distribution around the mean, colloquially known today as the bell curve, and Galton's application of it to what he vaguely called 'mental ability'. Here, equality lies in the fact that the incidence of individuals below corresponds statistically with that of individuals above. Idiots need to be few because geniuses need to be few, otherwise they can't be geniuses. This particular system of reciprocity and exchange is skewed by the values of the ladder of nature: geniuses, despite being abnormal, are still members of the ingroup because they are what the rest of that group aspires to or can even fancy themselves to be, whereas idiots are non-members because they are what the rest are fleeing from. Before Galton, there was a bulge at the bottom of the ladder: most people were quasi-bestial, unredeemable and idiotic. Now that the ladder is a bell-shaped curve of distribution around the mean, the bulge has simply shifted up to the middle rungs: most people are normal.

Of course cognitive ability testing features within the band of normal too, but the app on my smartphone is not assessment in its original incarnation; it is merely a trivial offshoot of that moral panic about idiocy which started with the rise of public statistics and continues today. In 1871 the official UK Census first began asking for the number of idiots or imbeciles in a household. This more or less invisible group thus had a vital role in the development of public statistics as a whole. A teleological world view in which individual intelligence plays a primary role forms the historical root of statistics in the human sciences in general. In such precise details we can see how that world view has been a massive force in class politics and social organization. The 1871 Census also took place at a time when the new long-stay hospitals were starting to fill with idiots, and compulsory schooling, just then being introduced, necessarily entailed a concept of the ineducable that would lead to the building of segregated schools. The same is true of the USA, where census categories implicitly overlapping idiocy with race.

In the UK, as the official Census introduced idiocy, Galton was starting to apply the bell curve to it. He adapted his theory of the mean from the Belgian astronomer Adolphe Quetelet, who had attempted to apply physics to society – a 'social physics' that would help adapt the common, species-wide definition of what a human being is to Locke's novel emphasis on the internal operations of the individual mind. Since both the theological idea of humankind as a 'whole lump' and the philosophical one of a generic 'rational animal' had proved inadequate, a new stability could be achieved with the 'average man'. The variables of individuals, said Quetelet, could be measured by referring them to a mean; here he was following the law of normal distribution which, though devised around 1800 as an arithmetical formula, had not so far been applied to the human realm. Quetelet, as well as suggesting its usefulness for collecting data on social variables such as crime, marriage, suicide, etc., applied it to people's physical characteristics.

The usual story is that Galton got the idea of measuring people's mental ability (he did not use the word intelligence in this context) from Quetelet's measurements of height. This standard account reflects another of inclusion phobia's schizoid reifications by ignoring what is in fact a clear historical dialectic. It presents the picture as static. Both actions, Galton's and Quetelet's, are presented as equivalent, since both occur within a permanent, unchanging biological realm of natural kinds. Height and intelligence seem to start out from the same place and therefore to furnish comparable examples. But the actions could not have been equivalent, because they were not two applications of one and the same principle. They came in a concrete historical sequence, in which the second took off from the first. Quetelet's mind ran: 1. There is an obvious natural fact (height). 2. Perhaps it can be described as a social fact, using the bell curve. Galton's mind, a generation later, ran: 1. Quetelet has described height as a social fact using the bell curve. 2. Perhaps the bell curve can be used to register as both a natural and a social fact something that has not so far been thus registered (mental ability). Height was a given fact of nature; but mental ability or intelligence – at that point in history – still was not.

Thus Quetelet did indeed come across the mean height of a population – if only temporarily (his finding could be falsified, and eventually was). Galton, by contrast, did not come across the mean mental ability of a population, he came across the *abstract idea of the mean* which he *then* cast in the role of mental ability. As for its concrete list of contents, that was his own personal choice. Therefore his theory of equal distribution of mental ability around the mean did not, could not and cannot get even as far as being falsifiable. It did, however, replace the lump with the 'norm', as the species marker to which the individual might once more be subordinated. As such, it formed part of an expanding artillery of social conformism and population control. With intellectual ability and disability, the individual becomes a number. The actual content of intelligence, prior to measuring it, can be whatever any Tom, Dick or Francis wants it to be; its claim to reality lies in the statistical mindset – there and nowhere else. Without the presupposition that the number of people at any deviation from the mean is equal on either side, intelligence as we construct it could not exist. The learning disabled person's lack of it is therefore a statistical artefact – a way of preventing them from being who they actually are.

There is a further striking difference between Quetelet and Galton. Quetelet pursued the principle of the mean because the value system in the back of his mind, an ancient one stretching back to the Greeks, told him that the mean is nature's ideal. A small person was as useful for clearing sewers as a tall one was for picking apples. Galton, in contrast, created a picture in which the ideal is not the mean itself but one out of the two possible extreme deviations from it. That is why it is justifiable to say that aspiration to the status of genius is a continuation of the medieval theologian's aspiration to angelic status. IQ and the normal distribution of intelligence, with all their temporal emphasis (as 'development'), hide the fact that they are still in fact a *spatial* and thus a closed, history-denying mentality, in Gabel's sense.

The extreme deviation at the opposite side of the mean came to constitute not merely a statistically neutral abnormality but *sub*normality, again a spatial concept. Deviation was the heartbeat of Galton's whole view of the human and social world, and of those who came after him to put the substantial statistical flesh on Galton's bare eugenic bones. And it was the *downward* character of that deviation that was the spinal column of intelligence. It exercised a gravitational pull on the upward deviation or aspiration, causing regression to the mean. Anxiety about this was their prior motivation, and one that we have seen over and again is a primary symptom of inclusion phobia. It is true that Galton and Pearson mostly used the theory of normal distribution as a weapon in the 'war', as Pearson warmly recommended, against racial outgroups; Laughlin, Davenport, and the American early developers of IQ testing were all likewise on a quest for racial purity. Be that as it may, the core target of morbid rationalism and measurement was and remains not race *as such* but inferior racial *intelligence*. It is necessary to keep repeating: intellectual disability is the farrago that feeds other forms of discrimination. In order to prevent the regular bindweed-like reappearances of psychometric racism and sexism, it is first necessary to dismantle delusions about intellectual disability as such.

It is worth noting here that although the early psychometricians espoused meritocracy, they had still not shaken off the traces of earlier religious and class-based forms of self-representation. Galton's first book, *Hereditary Genius*, from which the rest of his work developed, famously holds that 'high reputation', by which he also meant something like high social status such as gentility and honour, 'is a pretty accurate test of high ability'; and it is clear that even as late as this he meant the two were conceptually compatible members of one and the same class of things.[16] Moreover, although he exempted from this rule the old Anglican aristocracy whose reputations lay *solely* in their hereditary title, this was not because he was a democrat but because he was seeking equal parity for elites from his own rival nonconformist, but still elite, ancestry (Pearson's background was similar). It is not surprising, then, to find that the early eugenicists, meritocrats to a man with regard to people of normal intelligence, were at the same time obsessed with their own pedigrees. Laughlin, who established a Eugenics Record Office for mapping family trees, claimed descent from James Madison, while the atheist Davenport none the less claimed descent from God's elect, his direct ancestors having landed in New England in 1638 and their lineage going back (allegedly) to the Norman conquest.

This covert obsession with their own gentility was inextricably linked to their equal obsession with the family trees of degenerates, at the opposite end from the mean from themselves. Henry Goddard, lead inventor of IQ, laboriously traced the family tree of the Kallikaks in order to demonstrate that its members should be prevented from reproducing and thereby causing the general population to regress.[17] His detailed genealogy of the family came complete with (doctored) photographs illustrating the grotesqueness of its outgroup members and reinforcing the morbid rationalism of IQ, but in their layout they also bear a striking iconographic resemblance to the pictorial pro formas used by the heraldic assessors of Tudor honour elites.

Assessment by speed

Finally, morbid rationalism expresses itself in the increasing importance of speed. There are in fact three ways in which speed can be a value: fast is good, slow is good, or a mean is good. But today, just as intelligence is taken for granted as a natural kind, so is the idea that the faster we think, the more intelligent we are. The ideal that dominated Greco-Roman and early European thought was, by contrast, that of the mean: one could be too slow *or* too fast. Quickness came to be part of the core conception quite late, coinciding with the elevation of human reason. Nevertheless, the social history shows us a more mixed picture. In terms of everyday cleverness, the ability to think quickly had been valued in social and economic life for a long time. Words for slow had connotations of foolishness as far back as the Greeks and Romans. While the mean remained the ideal at a philosophical level, the development of the professions interacted with the increasing pace of socio-economic life. Likewise, the scientists of the early Royal Society referred constantly to the value of 'ingenuity', a term which at that time carried specific connotations of speed.

In church matters Luther and Calvin, both with humanist upbringings, were inclined to favour it.[18] Renaissance Catholicism taught that after death the soul has to pass through Purgatory; the very name signifies a cure for pollution. 'Purgatory ... is a realm of transition, of change, of making progress, of going from one place to another [on a] journey that will take many hundreds of years ... towards a heavenly home ... It conveys the new sense of urgency about time'.[19] Although the Protestants broke with Rome precisely because they objected to priests selling indulgences to speed you on your way, they absorbed much of the principle. Early on, the purgative escape from contamination had been spatial as well as temporal; Dante's protagonist ascends the mountain. Time would eventually predominate, leading to the idea of some people as 'backward' and contributing to the theory of childhood as a form of inner development. Seventeenth- and eighteenth-century Protestant educators like Watts, whose influence on our present cognitive cultures was as great or greater than that of the Enlightenment philosophers, were preoccupied with the idea of redeeming time on this earth. It was their emphasis on the scheduled mental 'exercise' of reason that formed the basis of their attacks on the 'idleness' of 'idiots and illiterates' who correspondingly threatened the social order.

The value placed on speed remained vague and unscientific until, with Galton's invention of the correlation coefficient, there came at the heart of it his intuition that speed and mental ability should correlate. Even then, this was largely ignored until the 1950s, when the invention of information science made it relevant. The whole premise of Artificial Intelligence, with its prospect of computerized thought overtaking the speed of computation in human brains, is descended from this recent reprise of information-processing as a characteristic of human cognition. It has ensured that speed is *constitutive* of intelligence. WISC tests, for example, in certain abstraction and information-processing skills, now score higher the faster they are completed. Galton's schema gave a whole new meaning to the assessment of certain people as slow. Their place on the curve of normal distribution means that slowness is not so much a negative value pasted on to some pre-existing disability but, rather, coterminous with it.

Such developments clearly belong in the material organization of a socio-economic life now dominated by speed.[20] Less than a generation after Galton, timed assessment would find a home in the scientific organization of labour known as industrial psychology. With the schizoid dehistoricization of time comes the takeover of the human personality by the commodification of time. As Gabel points out, this fulfils in psychiatric terms Marx's famous economic dictum that 'Time is everything, man is nothing: he is at the most time's carcass. Quality no longer matters. Quantity alone decides everything.' This applies to intellectual labour too. It reduces the person to an isolated particle fed into an alien system. The large majority, the ingroup of the normally intelligent and above, seems to have accepted this way of existing. Learning disability and learning disabled people are thus projections of its own alienation and suffering.

Notes

1 C. Nightingale (2012). *Segregation: A Global History of Divided Cities.* Chicago: University of Chicago Press, p. 32; *Times Higher Education Supplement*, 21 June 2012.

2 M. Nussbaum (2007). *Frontiers of Justice: Disability, Nationality, Species Membership*. Cambridge, MA: Harvard University Press.

3 P. Anderson (1997). 'Is measurement itself an emergent property?' *Complexity* 3(1), 14–16.

4 K. Smelik and M. Coetsier (eds) (2014). *Etty Hillesum: The Complete Works 1941–43*. Aachen, Germany: Shaker.

5 J. Gabel (1978). 'Rêveries utopiques chez un schizophrène', in *L'Evolution psychiatrique*, 1952, reprinted in Gabel, *Idéologies*. Paris: Anthropos, p. 315.

6 H. Laughlin (1916). 'Rating the several sovereign nations on a basis equitable for the allotment of representation to a world parliament', *Scientific Monthly* 3, cited in J. McDonald (2013). 'Making the world safe for eugenics: the eugenicist Harry H. Laughlin's encounters with American internationalism', *The Journal of the Gilded Age and Progressive Era* 12(3), 379–411. See also H. Brunius (2007). *Better for All the World: The Secret History of Forced Sterilization and America's Quest for Racial Purity*. New York: Vintage.

7 See for example P. Irwing and R. Lynn (2005). 'Sex differences in means and variability on the Progressive Matrices in university students: a meta-analysis', *British Journal of Psychology* 96, 505–524.

8 L. Wittgenstein (1981). *Remarks on the Foundation of Mathematics*. Oxford: Blackwell.

9 See for example L. Haynes et al. (2012). *Test, Learn, Adapt: Developing Public Policy with Randomised Control Trials*. London: Cabinet Office Behavioural Insights Team. See also G. Thomas (2013). 'No one can control for a sense of when 4-3-3 might turn the game', *Times Higher Education*, 7 February.

10 P. Monaghan and T. Birkhead (2013). 'Variety: the spice of life sciences', *Times Higher Education*, 27 June.

11 M. Donaldson (1978). *Children's Minds*. London: Fontana.

12 See Chapter 3.

13 I. Green (1996). *The Christian's ABC: Catechisms and Catechizing in England c.1530–1740*. Oxford: Clarendon Press.

14 T. Porter (1995). *Trust in Numbers: The Pursuit of Objectivity in Science and Public Life*. Princeton, NJ: Princeton University Press.

15 I. Watts (1811). *The Improvement of the Mind: Or, A Supplement to the Art of Logic*. London: Rivington, p. 150.

16 F. Galton (1869). *Hereditary Genius: An Inquiry into its Laws and Consequences*. London: Macmillan, p. 2.

17 S. Gould (1996). *The Mismeasure of Man*. New York: Norton.

18 M. Taylor (2014). *Speed Limits: Where Time Went and Why We Have So Little Left*. New Haven, CT: Yale University Press.

19 P. Shaw (2014). *Reading Dante: From Here to Eternity*. New York: Norton, p. 149.

20 P. Virilio (1977). *Speed and Politics: An Essay on Dromology*. New York: Semiotext(e).

8   Autism and its creation

A colleague and I, researching with families in a local government area that had adopted a radical inclusion policy, heard professionals use 'autism' occasionally of a small proportion of the children who were transferring to ordinary schools from a segregated one designated for severe learning difficulties. This was the 1990s, just ahead of the diagnostic explosion.[1] Under the circumstances we did not need to pay much attention to it, nor at that stage did the families themselves appear to do so. They used the label rarely, if ever, among each other. It was irrelevant to the most important things in the home environment. We took for granted the unconditionality of the relationship between parents and children, especially in a working-class community that shrank from the violence of naming.

If the world at that point had consisted entirely of these children, their families, friends, acquaintances and ourselves, there would have been no autism. Anyone in a sane frame of mind recognizes and knows *people* first. We know and recognize cognitive and behavioural patterns in them only subsequently, and only if we have been pre-programmed with a description of those patterns, which are often a product of morbid rationalism. Neither families nor qualitative researchers obtain their idea of autism from the person in front of them. They obtain it from something outside the person, from a fixed set of presuppositions that are nevertheless, in the long term, unstable and historically contingent.

Patterns are not needed in circumstances where the family is not engaging with the world beyond it. The reason why patterns are seen in a secondary social institution is because they are perceived to be needed there: say, for managing the autistic person's behaviour – even though the problem with inclusion phobia is self-evidently the behaviour of everyone else. What does the family want from secondary social institutions? Initially, for them to do the same: to accept the child, and moreover to accept him as Jake. Largely they do not. Sooner or later families stop expecting it to happen. Thinking it is impossible, however, or not being able to imagine it, or not knowing the simple things needed to make it happen, is not the same as not wanting it.

In a non-excluding political philosophy, the primary institution's values in relation to disability can extend to secondary ones such as schools, especially if they allow themselves to be led by the children in them, who absorb behaviour-patterning behaviour only gradually (and stressfully). At Jake's school, the first phase of including autistic children involved a Class 1, a separate room in the centre of the building where they spent some of the day with each other, though they also had places in various mainstream classes. Some of the latter children, noticing Jake was missing, would take the opportunity to go to Class 1 and tell teacher x there that his other teacher y wanted him in the ordinary classroom. They would then return with Jake and tell teacher y that teacher x had sent him. We observed the end of a class when the teacher and all the children had left bar one, who was just skipping out of the room when she noticed Jake's dribble on one of the desks, whereupon she dodged back, still skipping, to a box of tissues and wiped it up on her way out. Class 1 was later done away with. An inclusive primary school institution can sometimes resemble home, even within educational structures that are anxiety-driven overall. Where peer support was not forthcoming, this school eventually used person-centred planning with the other children, setting targets for their relationships with Jake rather than the other way round.

The family as the primary social institution is the last redoubt in the modern world where human relationships may be unconditional. The Roman 'family', for example, included tenants and slaves, who could inherit their masters' wealth, and through to the seventeenth century it would still have included servants and lowly or distant relatives; but in the modern stretching of social relations it has lost its status functions to wider institutions, and to national rather than local criteria. Hence the exposure and firming up of the idea of the wrong child, increasingly demarcated by the obsessive compulsions of medical and statistical research on the lookout for threats.

Inclusion phobia's most striking symptom, in any era, is the sheer range of descriptive characteristics it will attribute to the particular extreme outgroup that is its central obsession. The variability and arbitrariness of these characteristics are in inverse proportion to the unitary and fixed nature of the category they purport to describe. The onset is sudden. Ingroups are struck down with the new, pandemic mutation of an old virus. In the early twentieth century inclusion phobia's obsession with morons left no doubt about their clinical and biological existence, though we now only hear of them in street insults.[2] Anyone working in a professional capacity (leaving aside dinner-table chat about nice residential areas or good schools for the children) would agree that the idea of hordes of subnormals with borderline IQ roaming the nearby streets and threatening the future of the white race was a dystopian fantasy. Yet today, only with a different profile, we have hordes of people 'on the spectrum'. In this and the following chapter we therefore find ourselves going over some of the old features of inclusion phobia within what seems to be a new paradigm, which is in the process of occupying centre stage right now. The volume of segregated provision, funding, research, and public discussion that currently goes into autism provides a halo of justification for the demarcation of this new outgroup category. Is it just that clinicians of a century ago were primitives who made false classifications like moronism but that we make true ones?

Take the notion of 'quasi-autism': the persistence, in a minority of children adopted from East European orphanages, of features (not necessarily with 'cognitive impairment') that are 'phenomenologically similar' to autism.[3] No one is doubting in principle that environment may react back on an individual's biochemistry. But there is something spurious about how that similarity is presented. It encourages belief that the *psychological* category, as such, belongs to the realm of nature in the same way that a person's biology does, rather than being just one among many possible and equally soft-edged, cultural forms of perceiving others. Quasi-autism could equally be inferred from social deprivation, for example, and so *to* social class. What is there to stop this slippage? Rutter's concept in this sense just continues and projects into the future certain past notions of class idiocy; for instance, that of the head of the British Eugenics Society who in 1947 was claiming that 'the intractable ineducability' of 'problem families' simulates a 'genetically determined process'.[4]

Seventy years ago, the present description of autism was unknown. Just over a century ago, the word itself was unknown. And thanks to the specialism of history, which provides us with a general overview of inclusion phobia and its extreme outgroups, we know that one day there will be no autism – not because it has been cured or eliminated, but because our anxieties will have turned elsewhere. A historical approach provides no less valid an evidential basis than that of the psychiatrist or geneticist, and raises questions that must be answered before the latter can be confident that autism is not just another moronism. The current definition is hardly more than a generation old. Does this mean that some real subcategory of human nature existed in the past in an unrecognized state, and is properly recognized only now? (Hence all those headlines such as 'Was Michelangelo/Mozart/Marilyn Monroe Autistic?' in popular science columns, not to mention serious medical journals.[5]) That it did not exist in the past but does now? Or that it does not exist *even* now? The lists of ingredients and their definitive quality, such as it is, derives from a human consensus, which changes radically along with changing forms of social organization and associated anxieties. Although biochemists have to agree on where to section off a DNA sequence in order to call something a gene, DNA itself does not exist by consensus. A psychiatric consensus, however, sounds more like a political one; and at least politicians, unlike their psychiatric peers, know that agreements are always temporary.

The biological status of autism

To ask whether autism exists sounds scandalous. Brain-imaging technology displays it, geneticists are on the trail of its causes. Eminent professionals head research bodies that channel funding towards the condition that is their own expertise, backed by government and the drug companies. It is an accepted part of daily conversation. Phobic thinking creates a feedback between the secondary and the primary institution, which then enhances the profile of its target population. Lorna Wing, the 1981 re-inventor of Asperger's syndrome, is routinely described as a parent who happened to be a psychiatrist, but she was equally a psychiatrist who happened to be a parent. Families now freely talk about autism by name, sometimes pathologizing it in front of brothers, sisters and friends. Behaviour-patterning behaviour has invaded the primary institution of the family, and I myself would not venture to challenge its use in my everyday interactions with families.

The motive for experts to speculate about genetic causes was originally to divert blame from parents whom a previous generation of experts had demonized, by saying that their child's condition was caused by parental coldness in infancy. Nevertheless, the experts responsible for this shift have at exactly the same time changed the description of what constitutes autism beyond recognition. As with learning disability, then, it is not clear who we are talking about. The covering assumption is that the definition is right this time even if it was wrong the time before. But every generation thinks that, until it is contradicted by its successors. Wing, Uta Frith and Michael Rutter, champions of the definition currently in use, have seized on patterns of behaviour and/or mind that are (a) distinct from normal and (b) distinct from other abnormal patterns. Their initial aim, despite the evident empire-building it has involved, was to humanize families. However, what this certainly did not do was normalize those families. What the new definition of autism said on the tin was the admirable 'No more refrigerator mothers', but what is inside the tin has been a displacement of the pathology from the wrong mother to the wrong child. This was the only available direction for autism to take within the parameters of inclusion phobia, premised as it is on the prior and necessary presence in certain other people of that which is wrong, rather than as a pure biologist would conceive it, just different. Autism is just one more expression of the mind sciences' aspiration to be as exact as biology. The method is to use pathology as the means to establish a link between immaterial minds and material, bodily reality.

It is not the presence of biology as such that is the problem. For example, results have recently been obtained from a study identifying 'autistic' behaviour in mice – that is, certain behaviours that cause social anxiety when observed in human beings. Experimenters inserted a virus responsible for leaks in the gastrointestinal tract into pregnant mice, whose subsequent offspring were less social and exhibited repetitive behaviours. Once the mice's gut cells re-bonded, those behaviours diminished.[6] Moreover, it is possible that what is currently (i.e. transiently) classified as autistic spectrum disorder may indeed be the result of an interaction between 'biological or genetic factors' and dispositional ones, i.e. an 'enduring pattern of inner experience and behaviour that deviates from the norm of the individual's culture', as PsychCentral liberally puts it. Nevertheless, even if there were a physiological or genetic role, causal and/or interactive, for a particular set of culturally anomalous behaviours, it would beg the question of why and how that culture has swung round to a position where *it* in turn causes that genetic material to be highlighted, let alone sought: in other words for it to exist at all in any sense that would be meaningful or important for us.

The problem is not that bodily medicine thinks it has a role (and in any case, the mouse researchers themselves expect only modification, not cure). Rather, it is the presence of psychological categories within the experimental arena – as if, in terms of proof, they had equality of status with physiological realities. The listing of things that get to be called autistic is changeable and arbitrary; human DNA has been around for several hundred thousand years, the autism a few decades.

Moreover, to be anxious about those behaviours is a reflection on the ingroup's own. (If the authorities on comparative psychology are to be trusted, mice and other non-human animals do not experience disgust.) It is not Alex, measured as making the same smiley head-butting movement 2.4 times a minute, who suffers any anxiety about it; nor do the support workers who have gone to the local fair with him and who reciprocate with it as a visible gesture of friendship (intensive interaction, as it is called). No suffering is going on other than that of the non-autistic population touched by inclusion phobia.

Most autism researchers work from databases. They do not meet Alexes, and cannot therefore claim a knowledge of autism, let alone a workable hypothesis.[7] They are like traders fixing unpredictable future prices on a random pool of basic commodities whose poverty-stricken purchasers in Africa they will never meet. Many more research hours in brain imaging and genetics involve technicians than they do lead experts. On the one hand it is not the technicians' job to question the unfalsifiable hypotheses which experts present to them as given facts of nature; on the other hand, neuroscience and brain-imaging expertise entirely neglect to monitor the most basic element in their own field of knowledge, which is the actual relationship between mind and body.[8] It is often said by critics in the field of learning disability that scientists behave like God, but the problem is deeper, namely: not everything that says it is science actually is. And an experiment that incorporates psychological categories with medical explanations usually is not.

Brain imaging

One claim is that human beings have a dedicated brain function that attributes intentions to other people. Neuroscience calls this function Theory of Mind. Brain scans reveal it, since blood flow will light up specific areas where the brain is working harder. And it was precisely autism, the negative case (Mind Blindness, where the brain works less hard) that kick-started neuroscience's hypothesis about Theory of Mind.[9] The hypothesis that some people do *not* have Theory of Mind first established what Theory of Mind *is*, showing once again to what extent moral panics and outgroup formation are the driving force in refurbishing the normal. The autism that has defined mind-blind people, prior to their being subjected to Theory of Mind experiments, is a set of behaviours with a short-term historical existence, merely agreed or voted on by expert bodies, or prescribed by the most powerful mediators of research funding. Autistic people, in their role as creators of Theory of Mind, were only just pipped to the post by those other dangerously convincing mimics of fully human status, chimpanzees, illustrating the close connection between inclusion phobia and fear of animality.[10]

Theory of Mind involves various circularities, the first of which we noted in Chapter 3 and which medieval writers had already worried about. How can the understanding understand the understanding? The modern discipline tries to get round this by using psychology (lower case) to denote what is studied and Psychology (upper case) to denote the discipline that does the studying. Your discipline is not very secure if its subject–object relationship depends solely on a typographic convention. With autism this weakness is exacerbated, inasmuch as Psychology now adopts as its theory of mind the idea that Theory of Mind is a part of our psychology.

The second circularity is as follows. We say to our notional autist: you don't know what's going on in our (other people's) minds, but we do know what's going on in your minds, which is that you don't know what's going on in our minds, but we do know ...' etc. You are mind blind, we are mind seers. The very act of diagnosing mind-blind autism, especially as a device for segregating people conceptually and in social practice, itself exhibits an autistic failure to reciprocate.

The third brings us back to brain imaging. Here, the investigative trajectory – the history of the thought-process – runs as follows. (1) We are anxious about certain other people. (2) That must be because they are deficient. (3) Describe the deficiency as Mind Blindness. (4) Consequently, describe the capacity they are deficient in as Theory of Mind. (5) Therefore possessing Theory of Mind is normal. (6) Scan normal controls, i.e. anyone not already categorized as deficient, in order to establish where Theory of Mind is located in the brain. (7) Scan the brains of people already categorized as deficient to see if the region thus located is less active in them. (8) If it is, the scanning must prove a link between lack of brain activity and lack of Theory of Mind. It should be noted that (1) is preceded by an anxiety about ourselves; this explains how a ready-made, specific deficiency can always be at hand.

It would of course be completely absurd to take people already defined as autistic by a brain scan, subject them to a second brain scan and then say 'this (second) brain scan is evidence of a link to autism'. But it is equally absurd to take people already identified as autistic by a temporary consensus, subject them to a brain scan and then say 'this brain scan is evidence of a link to autism'. The association between autism and the brain is fortuitous. It is predetermined by the fact that you have available a particular facility for measuring a certain material substance, and that it just happens to be one which can be correlated with whatever immaterial, internal feature we think is important to categorize at that historical moment. In short, coincidence. Substitute bumps on the skull for blood flows in the brain, and you have nineteenth-century phrenology; head size, and you have Renaissance physiognomics; phlegm, and you have the ancient Greek theory of the four humours. All of these were ways of accounting for mental states. Critical psychiatrists call this the technology alibi:

> The mind is represented in the brain – the mind is tantamount to a set of behaviours – hence, all behaviours are represented in the brain – abnormal behaviours are still behaviours – hence, all abnormal behaviours have brain representation – hence, the fact that no brain representation can yet be found for mental disorders must be due to faulty techniques.

As these authors go on to point out, 'Finding something in the brain that might be related to the disorder under investigation would not prove the truth of the foundational claim placed at the beginning', so the sequence is deduced from an unproven assertion.[11]

Attributing significance to coincidence is a classic thought move in schizophrenia, and thus in inclusion phobia. In an unwitting acknowledgement of this, neuroscientist Chris Frith once described the 'luck' he had of being in the right place at the right time when scanning first came in, just at the moment when psychologist Uta Frith had started to wonder if Theory of Mind might have a dedicated brain system.[12] Let's say they have come home from their separate workplaces one day and are unwinding over a cup of tea. A thought strikes Uta: 'Let's call autism an inability to attribute motives and intentions to others. I wonder if there is a dedicated brain region for the ability to do so?' Chris replies, 'Well, at work we've got this new technique called brain imaging. If there is, an MRI scan will show correspondences.' On top of one unfalsifiable premise, that the mind is represented in the brain, comes another: that the mind, either as an invisible process or as reducible to an external set of behaviours, is an item in the natural world in the same sense as the material brain is, and thus that there can be a valid correspondence between them.

The biology community as such remains sceptical about the technology. The 2012 Ig Nobel prize for provocatively improbable research was won by an experiment designed to show how easy it is to obtain false MRI positives, which succeeded in demonstrating brain activity in a dead fish.[13] Meta-analysis shows that in the majority of reports on brain imaging, no attempt has been made to replicate findings.[14] It has also established that 92 per cent of investigations that scan brain areas anatomically have discovered something that is not actually there.[15] In almost half of published results only one scan is taken; consequently there is no control for the possibility of random fluctuations in blood flow or brain activity over the course of the experiment. The result is what biologists have called 'voodoo correlations'.[16] However, there is less than meets the eye in these criticisms. Their sceptical authors simply want better techniques. It will be done properly next time. They do not probe the thing they really ought to be sceptical about: that is, the prior assumption that an experiment using chalk and cheese simultaneously can be validated by pretending that two entirely separate orders of reality and two entirely separate methodological realms are one. Neuroscience has arrived at the point where it claims to be an explanation for absolutely everything, from everyday human behaviours to the highest cultural achievements.[17] But at that point it loses any possible significance. Neuroeverything leads to 'neuronothing'.[18]

Genetic research into autism comes up against similar problems to brain-imaging. Is a consensus-derived description of what does and does not constitute autism real in the same way that DNA is real? The description of autism is drawn from discussion and debate, whose roots lie in our anxious noting of behaviours, which can be added to or subtracted from the list at any point. Is 'from discussion and debate' the same sort of thing as 'from observation of the reactions in a pipette'? The correspondence between genes and mind, and the stable reality of the latter category as such, seem to have been verified by scientific method when in fact only the DNA has. The scientific status of categories of mind becomes accepted only through their being discussed in the same breath as material entities: innocence by association. Experimental verification of a link between two entities is easy if one of them is a dummy or catch-all. We are asked, furthermore, to accept a spectrum explanation: that across all individuals in a population, a psychological phenotype exists which shades from the abnormal into the normal, and that the genetic expression of these states likewise shades into the normal population. This is not a link, it is mere parallelism.

Linked to everything from anorexia to zinc deficiency, the autist provides a fantasist's field day for cognitive and behavioural genetics as promising as the moron once did. The point here is not to deny the very possibility that there is a genetic component to such differences, nor, conversely, that material causes do exist but lie somewhere else instead (the environment, for instance). It is rather to say that the ontological status of autistic spectrum disorder is in question when examined against the much longer conceptual history of the disorder that is inclusion phobia. This may appear to be a soft, 'cultural' criticism; but inasmuch as it *is* a criticism, it is probably more capable of empirical verification on historical grounds than the epidemiologically based claims of autism experts are on psychiatric grounds.

A very recent history

We can track the *lists* of autism's descriptive characteristics and how they have been taken apart and reassigned, ending in something like a 100 per cent blood transfusion. Finely distinguished sub-types of deficiency proliferated in the late nineteenth century, yet if individual characteristics that are autistic by the current definition can be retrospectively diagnosed there, the category cannot.[19] It belongs to recent history. In the first use of the term, by Bleuler in 1911, it meant obsessive withdrawal by certain individuals into fantasy and inner life, to the point of logic-denying hallucination. As Bonnie Evans has observed, this meaning was then largely conserved by the psychoanalysts who dominated psychiatry between the wars, and 'autism' and 'childhood schizophrenic syndrome' were being used synonymously as late as the 1970s.[20]

At the start there was potential overlap between autism and learning disability due to their shared relationship with development. At the time when autism still denoted a hallucinatory phase of schizophrenia, even the Freudians saw it also as a pre-developmental absence of logical reasoning: 'every infant begins its psychological life in an autistic state'. Thus there is a connection with Piaget, in that the psychoanalytic movement's 'understanding of autism was framed by a broader disciplinary-wide agreement that developmental psychology was a science that tracked the emergence of subjectivity.'[21] The obsession with autistic *children* followed the introduction of universal schooling, and like learning disability can be seen as an extreme outgrowth of earlier developmentalist anxiety about the reprobate status of children's souls. At the same time it provided the rationale for the description of autism in adults too.

From the late 1960s there was a move away from psychoanalytic approaches, with their focus on the individual subject, and towards epidemiological approaches imitative of those used for bodily disease. There was a revival of Kanner's 1943 call for autism studies to focus on externally observable signs rather than on guesswork about internal states. Some of those signs (e.g. difficulty relating to others, obsessive preoccupation with objects that stayed the same) were couched in terms still compatible with psychoanalysis. But at the same time they laid the ground for measurement and epidemiology to secure a grip on the definition. Morbid rationalism seized Rutter and others. Evans describes in detail how they went on to build an empire for statistical methods in autism research which was then internationalized by the World Health Organisation. It seemed to be the answer to Karl Popper's criticism that the social and mind sciences generally were mere outgrowths of medieval scholasticism. At last psychiatry would be a real science.

Because autism already had a place in developmental psychology, its re-assembly through number-crunching and a wholesale change of descriptive characteristics was not so difficult. Studies have increasingly employed autism as the core problem through which to understand other 'developmental abnormalities'. Reallocating it from associations of 'psychosis' to those of 'mental retardation' finally rid it of any psychoanalytic connotations. However, this reallocation was offset by the idea that it can involve non-retarded cognitive performances. The epidemiological turn, which found it as convenient to measure behaviours as to measure cognition, has thus drawn some of the attention away from the latter. Autism has therefore become perceptible in terms of general social interaction, rather than through the invisible character of individual parent–child relationships. If it is sometimes a matter of cognitive deficit, it is sometimes a matter of high cognitive ability, albeit within narrow areas. Wing's addition of Asperger's syndrome has enabled rapidly increasing numbers of children and adults to come under the umbrella.

We see here how a whole new outgroup paradigm can arise. In the evolution of psychiatric literature autism develops dialectically out of mental retardation (learning disability), partly overlapping with it but also expanding to cover new ground. Nothing illustrates this better than Asperger's own description of his eponymous condition. On the one hand it involves intelligence and 'a gift for logical ability, abstraction, precise thinking and formulating'; on the other hand, 'in the autistic individual abstraction is so highly developed that the relationship to the concrete, to objects and to people has largely been lost'.[22] Not only are these people *not* intellectually disabled, they star in one of the classic abilities of modern cognitive psychology – abstraction.

Let us track the movement in more detail. In 1980 DSM III invented a category of 'pervasive' developmental disorders, meaning abnormal development across a multiplicity of functions. At this point psychodynamic theories were being replaced as the central site of psychomedical cures in general by somatic, pharma-driven approaches.[23] At the same time, anti-social personality disorders were featuring more strongly. An atmosphere in which biotechnological prospects and social anxieties were recombining allowed autism to be completely recast. The turning-point was the 1987 revision of DSM III. For the first time it was supplied with detailed diagnostic criteria based on epidemiological models. It now became a lifetime condition, thus stealing more of mental retardation's clothes. With DSM IV (1994), autism became one of five discrete sections listed under that heading of 'pervasive developmental disorders', and with DSM 5 (2013) it has almost completely usurped the latter, one study estimating that 91 per cent of children with PDD could retain their diagnosis of autistic spectrum disorder from DSM IV.[24] Today, within the ASD category as such, the main subdivision is by *levels of severity*. Acquiring a measurable hierarchy on the ladder of nature is the final stage in autism's journey towards (pseudo-) scientific status, making it even more competitive as a diagnostic category with intellectual disability.

What DSM modestly calls its 'revisions' in this field are actually major upheavals. Of course DSM is merely a naming system, and does not assume a direct link from biological cause to label. But the revisions display the characteristically schizoid flips of inclusion phobia. Hallucinations having vanished from the list with DSM III, statistical research 'transformed the meaning of autism from a withdrawal into fantasy to an inability to fantasize'.[25] The change of context from psychoanalytic to cognitive and behavioural meant that over a single generation its content came to be the exact opposite of what it had started out as. The key moment had been Victor Lotter's novel list of twenty-four characteristics, drawn up in 1966. Taken individually most were not new, but their assembly together in one place was. To any expert of that time, especially one with the existing psychoanalytic training, they would have seemed a diffuse conjunction of items ransacked from previous studies of mental disorder across a wide range of unrelated categories. Since then, the victorious paradigm has regrouped Lotter's items around the 'triad of impairments' (though gradual, incremental refurbishments continue to be made). This illustrates Douglas' anthropological perspective on fear of contamination, which has at its core a 'circularity, such as supposing that a species must be anomalous because it is forbidden, and then setting up a search for its anomalous features'.[26]

What Douglas does not quite say is how historically concrete and precise this process can be. Our example demonstrates it. There were demands for the professional community to achieve consensus on a new list of symptoms. Lotter therefore asked it to 'agree on' definitional criteria that might lead to 'reproducible studies which would not be affected by the subjective judgments of individual researchers'.[27] This subjective fixity of purpose, spuriously representing itself as scientific objectivity, has enabled them to be directly attached to other conditions. The result is a proliferation of sub-sub-specialisms, such as 'Down's syndrome with autism'.[28] Now, it is certainly possible that alongside a chromosome difference some behaviours corresponding with those on the current autism list might be found; but that does not make autism a biological condition by association with trisomic ones. Rather, we can see in such extensions of the diagnosis yet another example of the obsessive-compulsive nature of inclusion phobia.

The rationality and the objectivity of the autism category come with hindsight. The items pasted together in Lotter's lottery have two things in common. One, they differ enough from the norm to make people anxious, and two, they are susceptible to measurement. Obsessive counting and anxiety about the unexpected are themselves autistic characteristics, and so Lotter's redefinition looks very much like a narcissistic projection of the ingroup's own pathology. Like the evolution of the idiot category described in Chapter 4, the evolution from Bleuler's concept of autism to the modern one is a move from temporary to permanent, from symptom to innate characteristic, from disposition to identity and nature. It is also a move from out of the ordinary to out of species. Hence the autism educator Ivor Lovaas, echoing Locke on the learning disabled changeling, describes his research subjects as people 'in the physical sense ... but not people in the psychological sense'.[29]

Concept and practice

Although in the modern era inclusion phobia has a single core outgroup, it retains a roving eye. Since all the historical evidence points to its being a disorder with a longer historical presence than any of the extreme outgroup categories it creates, we should assume autism is in a gradual process of transformation even now. This is best illustrated by practice. One specialist residential college I visit is subdivided into three different types of provision. After the MLD (moderate learning difficulties) department and the SLD (severe) department, I am shown into the ASD department. The people in there are similar to those in the previous two; just as in the latter, some come up to me, or smile directly at me, or initiate interactions (quicker than I do). On reflection I understand the rationale behind the separation. The first two groups are compliant, the third is clearly non-compliant. The distinction hinges on their oppositional nature.

This tells us something about the mutual reinforcement between phobic concept and phobic practice. A young person who in one establishment simply answers back too often may, if he moves to another, be reclassified alongside others who do not answer or speak at all. Institutional ghettoes reinforce conceptual ones, which in turn encourage more autism provision. Differential degrees of a certain behaviour – eye contact, mind-reading, polytropism etc. – may be observable among individuals. Sometimes we can even measure them. We are estimating, though, the performance of one particular behaviour. Autism is the name for a *collection* of behaviours and its corresponding identity, even though the itemized content of that collection varies even in the short term.

Why are traits *a*, *b* and *c* autism and *x*, *y* and *z* not? What has happened to the elimination of variables, which is standard procedure in the hard sciences? Autism experts have little to say about the problem. According to Frith, writing about Asperger's:

> At this stage, it is largely through detailed case studies that we can begin to understand the syndrome. Just as one comes to recognize a Mondrian painting by looking at other Mondrians, one can learn to recognise a patient with Asperger syndrome by looking at cases described by Asperger and other clinicians.[30]

There is something wrong with this analogy. The painter had to exist prior to giving birth to his offspring, his pictorial case studies. Frith however asks us to look at her offspring, her clinical case studies, *first* ('at this stage') – and *then* accept that they must all be the biologically determined products of a single progenitor category (Asperger's syndrome). The progenitor's existence is proved by the existence of its offspring, which proves they must be the offspring of that progenitor. Moreover, autism is so variable that it has the potential to be seen anywhere and everywhere, as its champions acknowledge. ('Show me an autistic person and I'll show you one individual person', says Frith's pupil Simon Baron-Cohen.) This seems like the projection onto other people of an excessive abstraction that is itself autistic. Whatever else it may be, it is a moral panic about an extreme outgroup. This raises the question, is learning disability just now, before our very eyes, metamorphosing into autism?

The term neurodiversity, first coined in the context of autism, is now being applied to learning disabilities in general, while the history of learning disability (under whatever name) is being rewritten as the history of autism.[31] Practitioners have started to use autism generically to denote a new binary with physical disability; a teacher tells me of a particular child I am about to meet, 'She isn't physically disabled, she's autistic', where previously he would have said 'she's got a learning disability'. Expressions of research interests in university departments now number more than ten times as many for autism as for learning disability; specialist education and social policy posts are advertised at higher salaries. Local education authorities that closed schools for learning disabilities and mainstreamed former inmates have subsequently opened new ones for autistic children. Learning disability thus shows signs of becoming an outmoded representation of the core outgroup, as the irrational mindset of inclusion phobia casts new roles for its paranoid dramas. In addition to the fact that not everyone in the new scenario is classified with low IQ, those who are not so classified, rather than being average, tend to be classified with high IQ. (This is especially the case in popular science writing.) If the dominant ideology were even semi-rational, of course, they would be distributed across the range of normal and above.

Autism's imperialist tendencies are illustrated by Amy, a ten-year-old with learning difficulties who gives me eye contact, makes friends, and tolerates and even enjoys variety in her routine. Her parents have trawled their local special schools including one specifically for autism. They send her there simply because they like its regime. In any case segregated institutions, subject to less external supervision (the people they deal with are not important enough), will bolster their roll with agreeable people who do not fit their label as often as they reject disagreeable ones who do. Amy has since been diagnosed with 'atypical autism', which now appears on her medical record too. Officially, atypical autism is a type that exhibits some symptoms and not others; but a subcategory like this is open season for the collusion between labelling, institutions, and provision. It expands the outer boundaries of autism, exposing it as an artefact of physical segregation. Build the concept and they will come.

What happens at the institutional level then feeds back at a conceptual level. When I was diagnosed with sarcoidosis, a usually harmless condition that mimics shadowing on the lung, my doctors did not tell me I had atypical lung cancer. A diagnosis of the mind, on the other hand, attracts absurd consequences. Epidemiologically generated evidence about the observed mind is as much a magic holdall as 'the unconscious' it replaced. A cognitive or behavioural pattern can be stretched in the observer's mind so far as to encompass almost anything, even (in Amy's case) its absence: clear evidence of inclusion phobia's schizoid nature. Compare Amy with Connie, an elderly lady who recently left the last of the UK's long-stay learning disability hospitals and moved into a community flat with large windows. She tells me how happy she is to be able, for the first time in her life, to see the moon through her window. By today's criteria she would probably not even have been diagnosed with a disability, though she spent most of her 82 years in the institution. In inclusion phobia's long historical timeframe, Amy's atypical autism is the learning disability that once denied Connie the night sky.

Autism and its critics

Evans notes the 'irony' of the label coming to mean the exact opposite of what it had once meant. But having done all the heavy lifting, she downs tools, neglecting to observe what this says about the arbitrariness of the act of categorization itself. Instead, she contrasts the 'enlightened' precision and 'evidence' of epidemiological studies with the research that used to 'speculate wildly about the thoughts of infants'. She locates a cross-historical permanence for autism at the level of its 'atypicality', transcending both approaches, when in fact it is a temporary and historically specific category imposed by inclusion phobia. Her detailed and objective analysis of the concept's transience is vitiated by her acceptance of the history-denying character of the epidemiological approach, which would have to be described as delusionary, in Gabel's clinical sense.

Other critics have tried to nail autism's socially constructed character. Like Evans, Majia Holmer Nadesan sees its present incarnation as an outgrowth of psychology's 'cognitive moment' around 1970. Unlike Evans, she regards brain imaging as wildly 'speculative'. Like most constructionist arguments, however, her critique inevitably suffers some slippage. We should avoid, she says, probing the '"truth"' or '"reality"' of autism; what matters instead is the discursive level, 'the view of the autistic person implied by these [speculative] assumptions'. Yet in the same breath Nadesan asks us to accept as truth – this time omitting the scare quotes – that a biological nature somehow accompanies the psychological category.[32] The critical element in her constructionist argument has an optimistic twist. Creating an autistic identity enables us to enrich our view of what it is to be human, and to celebrate that plurality. Thus its appearance in identity politics is not *only* 'divisive' but is 'simultaneously ... affirmative'.[33] If only to redress an existing imbalance, Nadesan seems to shade her argument in favour of affirmation, as do other cultural critics. It needs to be asked, though, whether 'celebrating' a separate autistic identity, even for such positive motives, does not also reinforce the opportunities for discrimination. Staff recruitment ads for residential workers feature the portraits of celebrated cases such as Beethoven, Newton and Einstein.[34] Once on the payroll, however, a carer may be so violent that people of this sort have to jump out of upper-floor windows to escape.[35]

The most basic conceptual issues are thus inextricable from those of social administration. The question as to *who* exactly are these people is bound up with the question *where* they are. How do they live? If you are Asperger's, you shall go to the diversity ball, even though your coach may sometimes turn into a pumpkin at midnight. Autism with severe learning disability, on the other hand, places you in the extreme outgroup, left behind for your own good. The proper place of optimism is social practice (the neutralizing of inclusion phobia), but the constructionist approach displaces it to the level of mere discourse – less of an uphill struggle. It offers optimism of the intellect, pessimism of the will. Celebratory social practices are commendable, but they will be piecemeal and take place in some inoffensive little paddock.

Nadesan's questioning of the word 'real' also needs thinking about. Being ambiguous about the reality of autism would not help in a court case against a carer who has really hit the autistic person they were caring for round the head. Nevertheless, being sceptical has its uses. A particular behaviour (say, hand-flapping) can be real in the sense that it is observable, but once we put several particular behaviours together, turn them into a category and then give the category a label (autism, for example), is that category as a whole real, in the same way? Philosophy answers this question in two opposing ways. The 'realist' school says that categories and species are universal, fixed entities, and that they exist quite independently of how we humans see the world. The 'nominalist' school says that when we assign real particulars to a general category, that does not make the category itself real: categories are ultimately arbitrary. Some have suggested that the nominalist way of looking at categories can sometimes be 'dynamic', in a feedback loop. That is to say, a condition that may have always been around, albeit uncategorized, comes to denote a tightly specified group of people simply by being talked about so much.[36]

Their nominal identity thus makes them open to recruitment. Sometimes, especially with Asperger's, it may even involve self-recruitment. There are always motives for voluntarily taking up an outgroup identity. In Tudor times, when the paradigmatic mental disorder was melancholia, there were notorious outbreaks of it among the gentry, especially those who had incurred the wrath of an absolutist state; by placing themselves offside, they none the less affirmed and celebrated an identity. An attention-seeker presenting with bodily pain will usually be rumbled as a case of Munchausen's, but the adoption of a psychological label, thanks to the fragile transience of its category boundaries, makes performance and self-identification much easier. It may even help restructure pre-existing individual personality differences. In an era of identity politics, people whose non-conforming personality would otherwise attract bullying or ostracism can find genuine refuge in a previously unavailable label.

The feedback loop may also derive from changes in forms of economic organization (for example, the rise of service occupations demanding social interaction), or simply from the plasticity of the brain.[37] Erving Goffman, the sociologist who first proposed the looping thesis, did indeed locate it in the material conditions of everyday life, by contrast with Foucault's discourse-based approach.[38] Another loop might be the establishment of segregated schools, colleges and services specifically for autism: people who do not communicate are confined to a sub-community of others who do not communicate, thus enhancing autism as well as extending it. Another autism critic, Ian Hacking, in a revival of Goffman's looping idea, simultaneously warns us that we are not to deny the reality of autism. In fact the more Hacking insists on the mobility of autism's category boundaries, the constant resetting of the menu of characteristics and the looping effect of social reactions to some eccentric individual personality, the more he feels obliged to insist also that he accepts its genetic or neurological associations. His nominalism thereby turns out, as so often, to be a covert appeal to realism.

How so? In fact, there is more than one version of nominalism. The original, medieval one was straightforwardly sceptical. It insisted on the arbitrariness of the categorizing process. But the more modern version, introduced by Locke and dominating the modern life sciences, is simply agnostic; it says that there may well be real categories and real species, it is just that our knowledge of them will always be provisional. Medieval realists had seen categories as real because God had fixed them once and for all, before the beginning of time. If agnostic humans cannot know how, we nevertheless bow down to the next best authority, the person with the most authoritative guess. Someone has to take charge of establishing reality, in the chaos of our ignorance. When nominalism was first proposed, that person was the Pope (hence his need for infallibility), but over the centuries he has been usurped by the expert.

Under pressure from the absolute presuppositions of present-day science, Hacking concedes a level of biological, cross-historical reality to the category of autistic spectrum disorder. In order to do this, he looks for the negative example that would contrast with his own. He finds it in the sudden arrival in the 1950s of a major new psychiatric condition called Multiple Personality Disorder, which then as suddenly disappeared. MPD was not real, he says, but autism is. However, if he had been writing in the 1950s, surrounded by equally absolute presuppositions (at that time psychoanalytic rather than cognitive) about the reality of MPD, who knows whether the pressure those presuppositions exerted on him would not have been just as strong? Would he not have cautioned that *that* condition was real, in a biological sense? If autism is a 'moving target', to use his own phrase, it is because inclusion phobia has moving targets. *This* is the unmoved mover, transcending all questions about the reality or otherwise of the conditions – the extreme outgroups – it creates.

Psychiatrist Lynn Waterhouse, while criticizing the urge to see in autism a single biological phenomenon, still maintains the conglomeration of symptoms *as* a conglomeration with a tidy existence of its own in some ahistorical nature of the mind, frozen in time.[39] Trust in biology cannot be dismissed in advance, but it is more than coincidence that we always leap to the general notion of biological cause *in respect of the current paradigm case*. The trailblazer at present happens to be autism rather than multiple personality disorder, in a world more irrational than that of Douglas' 'primitive societies'. At a level of reality beneath all the varieties of interpretation, autism exists. It must exist, because everyone says it does. Therefore *x*, *y* and *z* follow.

Hacking's conclusion is, rather, an ethical one. The more important question, he says, is: what are this person's strengths? Uta Frith also asks it.[40] However, what this seems to mean, for Frith at least, is *cognitive* strengths, such as an instant recall of bus timetables. Autistic people can be valued, but only by the thing that has damned them in the first place. In short, it is mere compensation (for 'difficulties in social relationships', as Frith terms them). In any case, this continues to leave out the most severe 'autistic' cases, the *extreme* outgroup on which exclusion disorder feeds, who would not know what a timetable was or be able to read one.

There can be other kinds of strength, even in the most severe cases, and these are exactly what the person's family and maybe a few acquaintances can already see, prior to pattern-making. They consist in the contribution someone's personality can make to a community by being there. This ethical point may look like simply an add-on, an 'ought' wheeled out to soften the 'is' of the disability itself. But the issue of people's strengths is epistemological as well as ethical. It can only be *merely* and *separately* ethical if the premise is that the people themselves constitute a separate entity, outside or against nature and society. Place them within an ordinary human community, with the non-restrictive support appropriate to them in present (transient) social conditions, and their outgroup identity and thereby the whole farrago may disappear. The half-pulled punches of constructionist and Foucauldian approaches, bypassing the due scepticism which is the initial stage of all new knowledge, retain a tacit acceptance of the category's essential reality. They share this with the medical models they otherwise refute. This only prolongs the social failure to see and accept what a person's strengths may be.

The most radical refutations come typically not from social critics but from within psychiatry itself. So for example clinician Sami Timimi calls autism 'a catch-all metaphor for a disparate range of behaviours that suggest a lack of the type of social and emotional competences thought to be necessary for ... societies dominated by neo-liberal economic and political foundations'. Yet this analysis too makes a partial reservation on people with 'more severe symptoms' and low IQ, which (he thinks) may indeed have biological causes.[41] The idea of biological causes is not necessarily false, but it is at best irrelevant to human community, and at worst damaging to all of us. No doubt autism's critics want to avoid taking their scepticism to the point of nihilistic posturing. But it is possible to envisage another goal entirely: to seek a sound knowledge base *somewhere else*, that is, in inclusion phobia and its concrete historical stages.

Notes

1 P. Alderson and C. Goodey (1999). *Enabling Education: Experiences in Special and Ordinary Schools.* London: Falmer.
2 G. O'Brien (2013). *Framing the Moron.*
3 M. Rutter et al. (1999). 'Quasi-autistic patterns following severe early global privation', *Journal of Child Psychology and Psychiatry* 40(4), 537–549.
4 C. Blacker (1947). *Problem Families: Five Inquiries.* London: Eugenics Society, p. 28.
5 See for example A. Leask et al. (2005). 'Evidence for autism in folklore?' *Archives of Disease in Childhood* 90, 271.
6 *New Scientist*, 16 February 2013.
7 A. Karmiloff-Smith (2010). 'Neuroimaging of the developing brain: taking "developing" seriously', *Human Brain Mapping* 31(6), 934–941.
8 D. Smukler (2005). 'Unauthorized minds: how 'theory of mind' theory misrepresents autism,' *Mental Retardation* 43, 11–24.
9 S. Baron-Cohen et al. (1985). 'Does the autistic child have a theory of mind?' *Cognition* 21, 37–46.
10 D. Premack and G. Woodruff (1978). 'Does the chimpanzee have a theory of mind?' *Behavioural and Brain Sciences* 1(4), 515–526.
11 G. Berrios and I. Markova (2002). 'Conceptual issues', in H. D'haenen et al. (eds), *Biological Psychiatry.* New York: Wiley.
12 C. Frith (2007). *Making up the Mind: How the Brain Creates Our Mental World.* Oxford: Blackwell; interview with Professor J. Al-Khallili, downloads.bbc.co.uk/radio4/transcripts/utafrith.rtf. Retrieved 14 October 2013.
13 C. Bennett et al. (2010). 'Neural correlates of interspecies perspective taking in the post-mortem Atlantic Salmon: an argument for proper multiple comparisons correction', *Journal of Serendipitous and Unexpected Results* 1(1), 1–5.

14 J. Ioannidis et al. (2001). 'Replication validity of genetic association studies', *Nature Genetics* 29, 306–309.

15 K. Button et al. (2013). 'Power failure: why small sample size undermines the reliability of neuroscience', *Nature Reviews Neuroscience* 14(5), 365. See also I. Chen (2013). 'Hidden depths', *New Scientist* 220 (19 October).

16 E. Vul et al. (2009). 'Puzzlingly high correlations in fMRI studies of emotion, personality, and social cognition', *Perspectives on Psychological Science* 4, 274–290.

17 P. Churchland (1986). *Neurophilosophy: Toward a Unified Science of the Mind-Brain.* Cambridge, MA: MIT Press.

18 R. Scruton (2011). 'Neurononsense and the soul', in J. Wentzel van Huyssteen and E. Wiebe (eds), *In Search of Self: Interdisciplinary Perspectives on Personhood.* Grand Rapids, MI: Eerdmans..

19 P. McDonagh (2007). 'Autism and modernism: a genealogical exploration', in M. Osteen (ed.), *Autism and Representation.* Abingdon: Routledge.

20 B. Evans (2013). 'How autism became autism: the radical transformation of a central concept of child development in Britain', *History of the Human Sciences* 26 (3), 3–31.

21 Evans, 'How autism became autism'.

22 H. Asperger, 'Autistic psychopathy in childhood', cited in McDonagh, 'Autism and modernism'.

23 D. Healy (1997). *The Antidepressant Era.* Cambridge, MA: Harvard University Press, p. 237.

24 M. Huerta et al. (2012). 'Application of DSM-5 criteria for autism spectrum disorder to three samples of children with DSM-IV diagnoses of pervasive developmental disorders', *American Journal of Psychiatry* 169(10), 1056–1064.

25 Evans, 'How autism became autism'.

26 Douglas, *Purity and Danger*, p. xiv.

27 Evans, p. 26.

28 N. Ji et al. (2011). 'Autism spectrum disorder in Down syndrome: cluster analysis of aberrant behaviour checklist data supports diagnosis', *Journal of Intellectual Disability Research* 55(11), 1064–77.

29 'After you hit a child, you can't just get up and leave him', *Psychology Today*, January 1974, cited in P. Chance 7(8), 76–84. Cf. Locke, *An Essay*, pp. 450, 571.

30 U. Frith (1992). *Autism and Asperger Syndrome.* Cambridge: Cambridge University Press.

31 See for example M. Waltz (2013). *Autism: A Social and Medical History.* London: Macmillan. See also R. Houston and U. Frith (2000). *Autism in History: The Case of Hugh Blair of Borgue.* Oxford: Blackwell.

32 M. Nadesan (2005). *Constructing Autism: Unravelling the 'Truth' and Understanding the Social.* London: Routledge, pp. 26, 125.

33 Nadesan, p. 209.

34 Advertisement for Brookdale Care (byline, 'Brookdale: Exclusively Autism') in *Community Care*, 7 October 2010.

35 M. Flynn (2012). *Serious Case Review: Winterbourne View Hospital.* South Gloucestershire Council.

36 I. Hacking (2004b). *Historical Ontology.* Cambridge, MA: Harvard University Press, p. 48. See also Hacking (2006b). 'What is Tom saying to Maureen?' *London Review of Books* 28(9); and Hacking (2006a). 'Making up people', *London Review of Books* 28(16).

37 J. Dupré (2012). *Processes of Life: Essays in the Philosophy of Biology.* Oxford: Oxford University Press.

38 E. Goffman (1961). *Asylums: Essays on the Social Situation of Mental Patients and Other Inmates.* New York: Doubleday; I. Hacking (2004a). 'Between Michel Foucault

and Erving Goffman: between discourse in the abstract and face-to-face interaction', *Economy and Society* 33(3), 277–302.

39 L. Waterhouse (2012). *Rethinking Autism: Variation and Complexity.* Amsterdam: Academic Press.

40 See for example U. Frith (1989). *Autism: Explaining the Enigma.* Oxford: Blackwell.

41 S. Timimi et al. (2011). *The Myth of Autism.* London: Macmillan, p. 5.

9 Autism in context

Jake has never spoken a word, and is dependent on other people at a basic level. It is a big leap from that to suppose that Jake or any of the other young people mentioned at the beginning of the previous chapter, who feature under 'autism with severe learning disability', think more privately or live more within themselves than any of the rest of us. They all know how to communicate their presence. They let you know what they want of you, and what they don't want of you. They know who likes them, who loves them, and who is frightened of them. They make sure to convey this knowledge to the rest of us. They are very easy to read, if you are prepared for the fact that they are reading you too, and very astutely; they all know instantly if you are not interested in them. Any 'incidents' with a professional carer are the result of this kind of failure, that it is to say, of the carer's autism. Actually they all give some eye contact too, though that may be because they all happen to have grown up in unsegregated environments. Jake's family accept the diagnosis of autism because of the social supports it brings with it, but they are still of the view as they always have been, after thirty-five years, that 'whether he can't speak or simply chooses not to' remains an open question; and if it is so for them, so it should therefore be for everyone else. In the theory of autism, however, it tends to be a closed one.

The history of inclusion phobia is the thread we must hold on to if we are going to escape from the labyrinthine question of what autism actually is. It is no good searching the past for primitive elements of the way it is defined at the moment. To get a proper fix we need instead to search for the separate contexts from which the current list of items came. And then we find that what seems like an ever-closer approximation to scientific truth is in fact no more than a change of direction in the interconnecting contingencies of economy, society, politics, and medical empire-building.

It would be naïve to think that just because there was no word for autism before 1911, the thing itself could not have existed. Researchers tapping into evolutionary psychology claim that something like monotropism may have developed in human beings as a survival strategy, a 'selective benefit' whose onset – albeit very early in the palaeolithic era – dates from after the beginnings of human culture.[1] Be that as it may, the reason our ancestors did not have a concept of autism was not because they failed to name it but because they did not need it.

The radical shifts even within the modern concept, noted in the previous chapter, indicate that there is not a firm enough base on which to make retrospective diagnoses of people from the past. Autism is defined as a deficiency in both intellect and emotions. The division between the two is itself modern and artificial. Perhaps the notion that autism is related to both is a sign that this divide is on the way out. Nevertheless I will follow this dualistic pattern for the time being, by looking first at historical notions of deficiency in communication and their political connection to heterodoxy and privacy; and second at the history of the emotions, at reciprocity, at kindness and sympathy (as precursors of empathy), and at the attribution of intentions to others.

Autism and totalitarianism

If the list of characteristics making up a category and their endless elasticity is a matter of choice – leaving aside the question: who has chosen, and for what motive? – then why is inclusion phobia's morbid, pattern-making rationalism in the precise form of autism necessary at this particular juncture in history? Both autism and its opposite poles (Theory of Mind, empathy, etc.) are historical contingencies because, like many theories about how the mind works, they have what sociologists call a latency function. Roughly speaking, everything must change so that everything can remain the same. Conceptual shifts help fixed structures to adjust to social change, but in so doing also maintain the underlying social *dys*function – in this case inclusion phobia, whose denial of history maintains the system as a closed one. Timimi describes autism as the result of a 'growing marriage between government and psychiatry ... rarely seen outside totalitarian regimes'.[2] To understand this, we need to look at totalitarianism more closely, beyond its conventional associations with Nazism and Sovietism.

Totalitarian political systems in the broad sense are alive in the democratic sphere. Forms of power extend ever deeper into the private realm of individuals. There are now few significant passages of human existence that have not been taken over and alienated as work, consumption or marketing time. The individual is constantly engaged, interfacing, interacting, communicating, responding or processing. The boundary between private and professional time and between work and consumption is elided; dislike of (superficial) change is an increasingly mistrusted and likewise autistic phenomenon, since the highest premium is on flexibility for its own sake. 'To always be doing something, to move, to change – this is what enjoys prestige'.[3]

The primitive totalitarians of the interwar years sought to produce a citizen who would conform to the state. Rather than pathologize rigidity, they instilled it. As Gabel points out, their own behaviour was autistic.[4] Nazism exhibited many of the behaviours Wing would observe in the people in her seminal Camberwell studies: rigidity of thought and behaviour; behaving as if other people do not exist; no response when spoken to; no response to cuddling; seeming to be in a world of their own; paying no attention to the other party; long replies to questions, spoken as if learnt from a book; voice sounding mechanical or monotonous; placing objects in long lines that cannot be moved; stereotyped movements; collecting strange objects; destructive and aggressive behaviour; screaming in public.[5] The psychiatrist Felix Guattari pointed to the 'genealogical continuity' between primitive forms and the current 'molecular' forms of totalitarianism that permeate everyday social institutions today.[6] It is an indicator of this change that the renovated concept of autism may be among them. Significant elements in its current version (deficiencies in social interaction, communication and adaptability, resistance to change) seem to match those of a totalitarian system projecting its own features onto an outgroup.

Present-day totalitarian democracies, as they have been termed, arose from the post-war ashes just as Kanner and Asperger were modernizing the label; political writers from centrist liberals like Isaiah Berlin across to Marxists like Slavoj Žižek have observed how democracy does not necessarily require or guarantee freedom. It gives the illusion of freedom through communication (the interpenetration of electronic flows), flexibility (the market), and horizontal social relationships (meritocracy). Its way of obscuring the fact that such freedoms and flexibilities are an illusion is to project their absence on to a small pathological category of people deemed to be incapable of them. Inflexibility, for example, either despite the market rhetoric or in cahoots with it, is typical of modern social roles, which people mistakenly think they acquire by choice. In autistic 'monotropism' this inflexibility is internalized, as part of a whole personal identity.[7] Thus, to use an anthropological distinction, it is not an acquired status (or in this case a failure to acquire it) but an ascribed status, i.e. one imposed by others.

Private thinking

Douglas, describing the way primitive societies apply social norms to 'anti-social' or 'interstitial' persons, refers to this as the imposition of an 'involuntary witchcraft'.[8] In the case of autism this is evident in the tensions between public and private reasoning. The idea of a private thinker existing in a private world has been identified as typical of autistic thinking,[9] but has also been a constant in the complex societies of the last two millennia. The historically specific trajectory runs from the social, externally observable characteristics of privacy towards inner, less obvious ones. So too has the accompanying social segregation of private thinkers on grounds of the dangers they pose.

It is often noted that the word idiot came from the Greek word *idiotes* – someone operating in an isolated capacity, away from the public arena of democratic decision-making. The word was not necessarily pejorative, though it sometimes indicated eccentricity. Later, in the Roman Empire and into the Renaissance, as we saw in Chapter 4, the same word could be used to identify someone inexpert in the key professions (the church, law, medicine), where the public arena was that of a social elite. In early modern England private often meant local, which could be a source of organized resistance to the state. Where there was a balance of power between the provinces and the centre, the accusation could run both ways. Hobbes constantly warned that private opinion was more subversive than public opinion, seeing no difference between it and heresy. Charles I saw Parliament as dangerous because it represented the needs of localities; Parliament's complaint against him was that, as an absolute monarch, he was driven by 'his own private reason'.[10] In short, private meant dangerous.

The modern division into public and private is thus an extended function of the political centre's gradual triumph over local power. The internalized, psychological element in privacy was an accusation designed to exclude people as early as the seventeenth century, when a local dignitary could be charged in court with being 'not familiar like a fellow, and that I did disdain every man's company' (a charge that sounds trivial enough until we realize that 'keeping company' was a civic duty).[11] If autism is private reasoning, inasmuch as it takes place beyond the ingroup, it must be seen in the broader political context of this history of privacy. Autistic people may be the ultimate nonconformists, but equally, nonconformists get to be called autistic. Private thinking is also politically heterodox, secretive thinking; and historically, heterodox thinking of any kind is by definition *un*reason. Power systems, whose centralized norms constitute reason, have always persecuted the secretive individual (while keeping their own sources secret). In Hobbes' time the monarch and his ecclesiastical henchmen could control public worship and prayer but officially could 'forbid none in private ... in our secret chambers'.[12] They were unwilling, though, to leave it at that. Their Maoist-style aim was for even 'the secret chambers of other[s] [to] be publicly reformed'. The chambers in question were people's minds.

When private reasoning had been a characteristic of the masses, neither personal nor political autonomy were conceivable. So what about the principles of democracy and liberal individualism that arose later? Their whole basis was the toleration of heterodoxy and dissent: the light of reason can only shine from within the individual if it is not induced or coerced by the centre. However, this was not the message which Locke, the main author of those principles, intended. Rather, it was: leave heterodoxy alone and it will tend towards homogeneity. In this way the private reasoning of individuals can fit in with normative, public reason well enough. Whatever human intelligence is, it is achieved by internal psychological mechanisms seen as common to all individuals. Consequently the residue of private reason that lies outside even this new norm, where those mechanisms are deemed absent or defective in certain individuals, distils down to a pathological minority.

From around 1700 terms such as 'the self' and 'the person', previously obscure philosophical jargon, gradually came to frame theories about how the mind worked, across nearly the entire population. They were a historical precondition for the very idea of awareness of self in relation to others (Theory of Mind).

The sense that private thinking is dangerous has been transferred to a small number of pathological individuals, in an era when for the rest of us that personal, internalized privacy has itself become thoroughly invaded.

Social interaction

Social interaction is by definition a restricted field: it can only take place between members of the group that defines itself as social, which over the span of European history we have been looking at has always effectively meant a more restricted group than that of the natural species. Our exclusion, by conceptual as well as physical segregation, of people deemed incapable of social interaction is only possible because our own historically arbitrary ingroup is defining the outer boundaries of what social interaction is. In current terms, 'socially interactive' means non-autistic. In a sane, inclusive environment it could be the other way round: when someone says of Jonny (in Chapter 2), diagnosed as 'autistic with severe learning disability', that 'it's an honour to receive his attention', this is not some self-conscious inversion of a norm which says that autism involves a failure to give attention to others, it is just a description of what it feels like to be in an ordinary relationship with Jonny.

There is a long tradition of similar circularities in previous theories of social interaction and communication. In anthropological terms, systems of reciprocity, the basis for social cohesion in general, often involve relationships that are unequal, between different social ranks or between an ingroup and an ordinary outgroup. However, we are talking here about an extreme outgroup: one that is shut out from the system of reciprocity as a whole. An observation of Aristotle's would resurface continually during the late middle ages and Renaissance. It entailed (a) a prior formula and (b) actual people to fill it. The formula ran: Were there a whole population entirely without honour or distinction of ranks, there would and could not be society among them. That is to say, such a population could not rule itself. Logically, then, any group lacking honour must be ruled by the rest, for its own good, and this must therefore be the group incapable of social interaction.

As for the characteristics of those people, they have changed over the longer term. The early modern honour society, for example, was partly a system for the sharing of information and thus of 'intelligence' in that sense. It defined social interaction, and therefore communication. But amongst whom? One had to be accepted for membership of the ingroup that was participating in that interaction; the ingroup at that point in history had not yet expanded to cover intelligence in its democratic or quasi-universal sense.

More recently, Theory of Mind internalizes a social system of reciprocity by presenting capacity for interaction as a state of mind in single individuals. Here too the system requires a negative in order to define it; therefore there must also be minds excluded from the system of reciprocity, on the grounds that they are individually incapable of it, as in Mind Blindness.[13] (It is worth noting that Frith's mentor, Hans Eysenck, cut his psychiatric teeth on testing for introversion, whose chief feature was similarly a tendency towards absence of social interaction.) Anthropologists see internalization and the attribution of mental states in general as a 'cultural function' of reciprocity, involving 'spiritual mechanisms' in the receipt or bestowal of esteem.[14] Viewed in this light, a diagnosis of autism is simply the removal of esteem as such, rather than a removal of the esteem accorded to some other referent. That is why we often extend it as an insult (colloquially but not always in jest) to anyone we take a dislike to, who fails to cave in to our demands, or simply doesn't talk a lot.

Another aspect of social interaction in the early modern era was 'conversation'. At the onset of the period this word entered the general set of Western life-skills as *conversatio*, the precise technical term for a capability that was confined to an intellectually skilled humanist and philosophical elite. The Reformation subsequently established ability to communicate as key to promoting its cultural transformation: a practical and self-conscious schooling in new forms of politeness. One took turns at civilized discussion about topics which might otherwise elicit dangerously conflictive opinions about religion or politics. 'Polite' conversation – that is, polished, clean, free from the contamination of difference – *was* conversation as such. The masses were as much impaired in this respect as they were in the intellectual capabilities discussed in earlier chapters.

Social history, however, and the necessities of commerce, had got there before the elite. Large numbers of people were expected to deliver a decent conversational performance in their everyday dealings, even at an inferior social level. Middling citizens' talk had to be backed up by a presentation of self and an awareness of how others might respond to them. As the author of a seventeenth-century handbook on retailing noted, 'honesty' without 'wisdom' was 'unprofitable'. An honest reputation (petty bourgeois honour) also required the small talk (petty bourgeois *conversatio*) that would enable a draper to do business effectively. 'Without this, his other qualities will not help him ... It cannot but be distasteful to any man, coming into a shop, when he sees a man stand as he were drowned in phlegm and puddle.'[15] On the contrary, in 1635 as in 2015, he should expect to be looked in the eye, smiled at and exhorted to have a lovely weekend. Only this morning, before sitting down to write, I passed a sign in a shop doorway: 'Sales assistant required. Must be bubbly.' It is just that today, when services are the archetypal occupation, the way we medicalize the dull or incommunicative ('phlegmatic') outgroup has become more precise: a further corroboration of Douglas' insistence that our conceptual apparatuses for preserving against contamination are rooted in the division of labour.

Kindness, sympathy, empathy

Closely associated with social interaction, communication and conversation is the autistic person's famous lack of empathy: an emotional rather than a cognitive deficit. Here we need to be careful. It is too easy, playing the game by the rules of a historically contingent binary between intellect and emotion, to dismiss 'emotional intelligence' and its absence as involving the same kind of phobia and morbid rationalism as the cognitive kind. In practice at least, educational or group psychotherapy routinely consists in helping people with their personal interventions rather than passing judgment on them or segregating them. Yet the choice of noun is unfortunate. There is consequently in the work of Baron-Cohen and others a whole know-your-own-EQ business with autism at the bottom of the ladder.[16] Moreover, the historical and investigative trajectory of pioneers in emotional intelligence shows a direct link back (just as the cognitive variety does) to prior anxieties about its absence in developmental disability and autism.[17]

Practice and personal interventions aside, all *general* or theoretical talk about emotions, as about intellect, is a form of ingroup self-representation. Correspondingly, there is a concrete 'historical economy of emotions' in which each society commends some and taboos others.[18] These emotions have their own place on the ladder of nature. Whereas human intelligence and reason constitute an ascent on the ladder towards being one with God the all-knowing, emotions ascend towards God the all-loving; people demonstrate how far up the ladder they are by the way they respond to their fellows. In this we can trace long- and medium-term shifts of meaning, and their relationship to the social structures of each era; hence, rather than meet general talk about emotions with an equally general theory of power, we can use historical knowledge to intervene in changing present structures, beyond just making a virtue of the autistic person's marginality.

It is lack of historical specificity that preserves the negative status of outgroups, because it obscures the primary role played by inclusion phobia. Empathy is the latest in a successive set of supposedly descriptive but actually normative terms for human interaction. These terms differentiate among individuals, create outgroups and ascribe values. Their normativity is hidden because otherwise it would expose the inequalities involved. Empathy – the concept, the discussion – is a historically specific phase in the longer-term setting of conditions by which human beings are individually and collectively sorted into their position on the ladder of nature. Before empathy, in the eighteenth and nineteenth centuries, there was sympathy, and before that, kindness. Historians have tended to conflate all three, with only a few token nods to period; to override specificity in this way is to encourage the assumption that empathy is natural, when in fact it is a modern invention.

On the one hand, the medieval 'kind' (noun) was what we now call the species (hence 'mankind'). On the other hand, the adjective denoted a personal quality that went with nobility and gentility. A gentleman should relate to everyone else as equals at one level (God has created all human souls in the same condition) even if he treats his inferiors with brutality at another (social hierarchies are natural and have to be enforced). If with the privilege of hindsight we can see the self-contradiction in this way of relating to other human beings, it goes with an inability to see the hypocrisy in our own. For example, we tend to take for granted the idea that there can be good motives for segregating people, but either the community includes the autistic outgroup or it does not. At least if the sixteenth-century outgroup, the hydra-headed multitude of social inferiors, was constantly deemed 'no better than brute beasts', it was only metaphorically. In everyday social terms, kindness meant generosity to one's elite peers and particularly to friends, but also courtesy towards human beings in general: that is what was meant by the phrase *noblesse oblige*. Kindness in this latter sense was proof of one's honour. So what about unkind people? Since concern for others was a property of the species as a whole, the only reservation on species membership had to be about people lacking such concern. These were the real emotional monsters. This is what Hamlet meant when he called his fratricidal uncle 'a little more than kin and less than kind'. Unkindness was close to psychopathy.

By the eighteenth century kindness was giving way to sympathy as the central concept, notably in David Hume and Adam Smith. (It broadly overlapped with 'fellow-feeling'; again, it is not actual labels that are at issue but the characteristics describing them – a century later George Eliot was using 'sympathy' to mean something much closer to modern empathy.) They argued that we should treat all human beings with a degree of equality in an everyday social sense as well as in a theological one. For them, sympathy described a human being's inner, psychological motives as much as an external social obligation. The principle of hierarchy remained lurking in the background, however. The source of sympathy was now self-interest; it was no longer a religious motive but a mental operation. I myself am at the centre of my concerns, but there is this mechanism in me that ripples from here through to family, then to social peers, then to country and race and finally to all human beings, in increasingly diluted form. I resonate with others, while remaining within the enclosed and private property of my 'self'. Smith explicitly refutes the suggestion that this mechanism should enable us to understand someone else's suffering by getting inside their head. Sympathy is not empathy but a reflecting device. Its opposite is disgust. For Smith, the non- or quasi-human outgroup is no longer the multitude, or at least not the broadly middle-class sector of it or even the skilled artisan. Instead, he instances the 'contempt' and 'detestation' to which 'idiots' (who probably still include unskilled labourers here) are naturally subject.[19]

To be incapable of sympathy was again something like psychopathy, deliberately ignoring the suffering of others because of the slightest inconvenience to oneself. Hume tries to imagine someone who would step on another's gouty toes as he was walking along the street, just because they were softer than the paving stones.[20] Being incapable of sympathy towards creatures who qualify for it is abnormal ('monstrous'). And therefore being incapable of sympathy towards creatures who are incapable of sympathy towards creatures who qualify for it must be normal. Rather than being just a ripple at the furthest edge of the pond, they are tipped into some other, non- or quasi-human category. That schizoid relationship between placing people out of the natural species or 'human kind' and *being* kind was thus continued by the idea of the person incapable of sympathy.

The idea of people incapable of empathy takes this further. For example, Baron-Cohen's idea of shading, that all of us are autistic to some degree, is simply Smith's social 'ripple effect', internalized as a hierarchy of individual competence. Fail to know what is going on inside someone else's head (say, your line manager's) and you stand in danger of being denounced as autistic just as in primitive totalitarian societies your insistence on privacy might get you denounced as an anti-party element. Even as it shades off into trivial insults of this type, a diagnosis of autism is thus what Girard calls a 'denunciation'. The scientific and the trivial everyday usages of the term lie on a single continuum that tracks Exclusion Spectrum Disorder, so to speak. The insult does not *derive from* the diagnosis but arises *simultaneously* with it, and *reinforces* it. Bleuler, even as he was coining the word autism, also observed this novel condition in fellow-experts opposed to his new theory. Just as we saw in Chapter 5, insults sometimes contribute to the making of classifications and diagnoses rather than coming after the event.

Differences between the three historical types are none the less evident. Kindness involved recognizing, if not how another person suffers, then at least *that* they suffer.[21] Psychiatrists have acknowledged that empathy, by contrast, may involve deliberately ignoring suffering. A torturer like Winston Smith's interrogator in *Nineteen Eighty-Four* has to be empathetic in order to see what will be the most painful thing for his victim.[22] One can be cruel to be kind, but one can be empathetic to be cruel. Baron-Cohen warns against taking absence of empathy to indicate an equivalence between autism and psychopathy; but once he had posited the general notion of someone in whom empathy is absent, that discussion obviously became too good an opportunity to miss.[23] The terms empathy and autism, along with the concepts they referred to, were coined within a few months of each other around 1910. Just as the notion of intellectual disability was intrinsic to that of intelligence (neither could be conceived without the other), there is an element of cruelty in empathy because the latter owes its existence to that equally modern but opposite, 'autistic' trait that hinders the species development of the desirable trait and thereby places the autistic person *out of* kind. In this sense, the very existence of a concept of empathy stems in part from a positive lack of kindness.

What seems to underlie the historical shift from kindness to sympathy to empathy, then, is the social codification of our reactions to supposed suffering in others. That which evokes kindness, sympathy and empathy in the observer can also evoke fear and phobic disgust. Suffering – in this case, apparent suffering – contaminates. It evokes fears of mortality. The ambivalence surrounding kindness, sympathy and empathy equally – the indecisiveness as to whether to include or exclude, or to try to do both at the same time – is a reflection of this and represents two sides of the same coin. To ask who they *exclude* is inextricable from the question of who they *produce*, as their own particular monsters.

In practice, empathy is as hard to pin down as its polar opposite.[24] As well as being that which is lacking in the private thinker, it is also an *invasion* of privacy. Financiers, priests, management consultants, feminist support groups, bullies, humanitarians, cold-callers, psychiatrists, waiters (to name but a few) – all of us are called upon to mobilize our empathy, as an operational tool for achieving our ends. Critics have noted the multiplicity of meanings of empathy, and its potential use as a weapon of the powerful. One kind of critical response, as with intelligence, is to substitute a 'good' definition for a bad one: seeing it, for example, not as stepping into someone else's shoes but as a permanent openness to affective experiences with each new individual encounter.[25] This is close to the way Jane Austen insisted the word 'nice' should be used, to mean responding appropriately to others by differentiating among their emotional states and understandings; even as she wrote, she realized that this would inevitably be swamped by over-general usage. As with intelligence, there is a lesson to be drawn: if you say the idea of empathy is a social construction, you cannot then lay down your own alternative laws for its use and expect to be obeyed. Anyone can do the same, and they will often be more powerful than you.

Autism and reciprocity

Social codification of our reactions to suffering returns us to the theme of reciprocity: this time, emotional reciprocity. With sympathy, we noted how Hume's monsters are incapable of reciprocating and thus they exhibit the ultimate in selfish egoism; they contravened the principles of a society whose own basic premise of sympathy in fact derived from self-interest. Hume distinguished egoism and self-interest from each other. The egoist who would step on another's gouty toes for their own trivial comfort is taking the prevailing ingroup mentality too literally, exposing its core principle of ethical self-interest for what it actually is by taking it to extremes. With empathy, the principle of reciprocity produces similar contradictions. There is a covert connection between the empathetic norm and its autistic opposite. To expose it, we must separate the question of who is designated as incapable of reciprocity from that of who actually suffers. People perceived as autistic do not suffer from their autism, though they may sometimes suffer from the reactions of other people. The empathetic (normal) ingroup, however, clearly suffers from the anxieties involved in their inclusion phobia, otherwise the autism category would not exist. We might say that autism is a delusion of that phobic state in the rest of us.

Autism is thus not the opposite of empathy but its doppelganger. Any failure to reciprocate is the *ingroup*'s failure to reciprocate, which expresses itself in allocating that failure to a category it casts as the outgroup. The fact that emotional states are attributed to non-human species less grudgingly than intelligence means that evolutionary psychologists have found empathy not just in chimpanzees and dolphins but in all mammalian species, including rats.[26] A creature incapable of empathy is not only non-human but also, it seems, not even mammalian. The bizarre idea of allocating such a place in nature to certain people arises from the state of mind suffering from inclusion phobia.

One criticism has been that a focus on lack of social interaction encourages the comparisons between autism and psychopathy; the focus should be instead on monotropism and stereotypy. Baron-Cohen responded to this challenge by classifying autism as characteristic of a 'systemizing' mind.[27] Systemizing provides a less pejorative alternative to psychopathy, as the opposite but still negative pole to the positive one of empathy. The insistence on identifying excessive systemizing as an autistic disorder seems itself to be an example of excessive systemizing. One obvious defence against this type of criticism is that the concept is epidemiological, denoting a statistical spread of behaviours and characteristics rather than a watertight classification of individuals. Nevertheless, once the concept gets entangled in administrative practice, the sharp demarcation of extreme cases, suggesting membership of a separate kind, results in segregation. Putting people (and particularly children) who supposedly do not communicate with others who do not communicate then grows them into quasi-human or monstrous roles which thereby exclude them from ordinary life. In this action, it is not clear who is the autist. Is it the people observed, or is it the observers?

Experimentally, the normative characteristics of empathy, just like intelligence, are modelled by those of the relevant expert. Take contagious yawning. As this is assumed to indicate empathy, might it be observed less in autistic people?[28] The experimental method is as follows. (1) Put certain behaviours and characteristics together in a list, omit others. (2) Call them autism. (3) Ask yourself whether a lower than average rate of responsive yawning might be added to the list. (4) Using non-autistic controls, study some children already allocated to the autism category. (5) Discover that they yawn less. (6) Put diminished responsive yawning on the list.[29]

This circularity is reinforced in the unequal exchange between observer and observed. When researchers observe their own behaviour, they find that they themselves yawn *more* than average. One experiment has found a correlation between people's sensitivity to yawning and their occupations; less yawning was observed in systems people such as engineers, more in members of the empathetic or 'caring' professions, among whom the psychologists devising the experiment numbered themselves.[30] The sole conclusion that can be drawn from this experiment, since it follows from a definition of empathy both determined by and exemplified in the experimenter, is that people who empathize more empathize more (nice people are nice people). All it indicates is that their starting criteria, presuppositions and entire conceptual apparatus belong to a temporary ideological standpoint that denies the reality of its own provisional character, exactly matching Gabel's description of social schizophrenia. This kind of solipsism, like those involved in intelligence, can even be acknowledged and justified within the system of knowledge itself – for example, in experiments that describe empathy and contagious yawning as an instrumental tactic for the bonding of ingroup self-interest through exclusion.[31]

Autism and gender

Along with privacy and some of the other features of autism, systemizing also involves gender, which throughout history has been a central prop in the categorizing of the emotions. Baron-Cohen refers to autism as the state of the systemizing 'extreme male brain'. Leaving aside his usual epidemiological caveats (it does not predict the behaviour of individual men), we can see how this helps to feminize normalcy. This is in keeping with the successes of liberal feminism, and the arrival of women in areas of life previously closed to them. It also recuperates or marginalizes more radical feminist ideas in the interests of a social order that continues to be run overwhelmingly by men. The successes can be seen as patriarchy's takeover and application of qualities that previously belonged to a private sphere dominated by female agency. Men have to acquire feminine characteristics if they are to stay in the driving seat.

There is a long historical pedigree, worth briefly illustrating, to Baron-Cohen's pathologization of the male as a route to maintaining patriarchy – typically by giving the impression that a power relation is being altered when it isn't. A well-known literary example is The Wife of Bath's Tale. Chaucer offsets the lively autonomy he has attributed to her in The Prologue by giving her a dubious story. An Arthurian knight rapes a woman and is condemned to death. The court ladies plead for a chance to re-educate him instead. They set him a test: he must answer the question, 'What is it that women want?' His reward for getting the answer right (women must be 'sovereign' over their partners) is that he gets the girl, a new and beautiful one, and retains his position at court – while the women fade back into political anonymity.

A century and a half later came the monarchy's call for infants of the nobility to be reared in an exclusively female setting, far from the rough male members of their clan. Adversarial men were not good role models for the Tudor regime's new social elite; virtue and excellence were now to be identified not with personal honour but with the obedient intellectual ability that could help run a centralized administration. There were ambiguities about class and gender in this call. The phrase 'new man' denoted pejoratively a member of the ruling elite who was low-born, such as Thomas Cromwell; but it also denoted a Puritan who believed himself to be regenerate and in grace. Being adversarial, in the sense of doing in private what the authorities banned, was castigated as 'feminine'[32] – even as the new man's espousal of (intellectual) obedience and grace over martial virtue covertly feminized him, helping him towards greater subtlety in his management of others and thus furthering his career. Women, while serving their turn at this discursive level, remained in their own private boxes.

Later still, the radical feminism of the Victorian era offered a fundamental alternative in the way human beings behave towards each other; the caring or nurturing values of maternal love were presented as a challenge to dominant patriarchal values. Yet a wedge was easily drawn between this and the eventually successful movement for political emancipation. Women on the whole only needed the nurturing image they already had of themselves to be confirmed;

men, as critics of the time could already see, needed softening up so that they might become more obedient to power at the same time as being more capable of wielding it.[33]

Applying these historical parallels to autism, we can see that if autism is the extreme male brain, this very proposition is itself a product of patriarchy. Baron-Cohen's feminization of normalcy and normalization of (liberal) feminism go hand in hand with his obsessive codification and labelling of the residue of pathologically private individuals. Today's managerialism has not only let women in, it has (it is said) applied the image of the good girl who sets a moral value on completing her work neatly and on time to both sexes indiscriminately, as a behavioural norm.[34] It disapproves men's tendency to go off on private trajectories of their own. At the same there has been an explosion of talk about interpersonal skills and emotional literacy; 'awareness of self in relation to others' has been elevated to a behavioural norm, an additional item on the list of species-defining human characteristics. These qualities, also necessary for management, are deemed to be female, by contrast with the typical qualities of the male who simultaneously wallows in and buttons up his private thinking. It should therefore come as no surprise – and is entirely in keeping with a schizophrenic logic – for the biological roots of autism to be sought on the Y chromosome.

Learning disability versus autism

Much of what we have looked at in this chapter features characteristics that apply to the whole of the so-called spectrum and thus take us some way from learning disability. The link between the features of low IQ autism and those of the rest of the spectrum, however, remains tenuous. In this sense the learning disability paradigm may not so easily be shifted; while one is no less an invention than the other, one is no less deeply embedded than the other.

In primitive totalitarian societies absence of empathy was encouraged because people's relationships and communications were ideally not with each other but with the state. Rather than communicate with others, one informed on them. Now, empathetic communication is insisted upon to an equally stifling degree. 'We know how you feel. We feel it too', as Sky TV's ads put it, while late capitalism's service economy demands empathetic personal skills that lay dormant when the typical proletarian task was to dig carrots or weld the same spot at an assembly line ninety-six times a day.[35] It is not surprising, therefore, that we should offload their absence on to a small minority of others. Yet it is not so small. 'Autistic' in colloquial usage often just means selfish, and if empathy is good for business it can still be missing in the businessman. To be rich, you must be monotropic, shut out distracting images of poverty, and maintain secrecy about the billions of dollars in your private bank account, at same time as using empathy in advertising and research to invade and capture the deepest privacy of our inner lives. It demands from us empathy on the job while urging us to feel free to be selfish as consumers. These shifting and contradictory terminologies feature in the successive regenerations of modern political and social organization. Autism did not enter ordinary discourse until a generation ago. Nor did empathy, as the key attribute in successful social functioning. Where once it was an esoteric term in aesthetics (which is how even within my own adult lifetime I came across the word for the very first time), empathy is now on everyone's lips and even stands at the core of a 'transnational politics' championed by prime ministers and presidents.[36] Is it then, just a fashion, rather than a paradigm?

We seem to have arrived at the point of saying that if autism did not exist we would have to invent it; yet in the long historical run the same is true of learning disability. All the refurbishments of the autistic personality indicate that empathy could not exist without it. Undermining the rigid separation of emotion from cognition in the modern era, autism and learning disability along with empathy and intelligence are united by notions of development and developmental disorder. Piaget's 'moral judgment', which referred to a child's affective development, already looks quite like what we now call empathy; it supposedly marks the transition at which the child begins to interact and co-operate with equals and learns to take into account the role of the other – an ability 'to see the same data from more than one point of view'.[37] Just as childhood is in cognitive terms a state of temporary idiocy, then, it is also, in emotional terms, a state of autism. (This is a view so deeply embedded that it may seem very strange when one points out the ethical perceptiveness and intentions of even very young children.[38])

Failure to develop moral judgment looks very much like the thing we refer to as adult autism. What, for Baron-Cohen (apart from political correctness), stands in the way of calling these people moral defectives, as we did certain people a century ago when we locked them up in the same places as people with learning disabilities and hardly noticed the distinction? If empathy is the supreme moral characteristic, then autists cannot be moral beings any more than people with learning disabilities can be rational beings, and are thus out of kind. And so in trying to pick a rational way through the shifting historical contingencies that are taking place before our eyes, in terms of *both* autism *and* learning disability, we continue for the time being to come up short against inclusion phobia and its most impenetrable symptom: the delusion that a certain social ingroup, however large, is the natural species. An awareness of this delusion is what provides the *terra firma*, the reliable knowledge base, for historical research and for social research and practice.

Notes

1 P. Spikins (2009). 'Autism, the integrations of "difference" and the origins of modern human behaviour', *Cambridge Archaeological Journal* 19(2), 179–201.
2 Timimi, *The Myth*, p. 5.
3 J. Crary (2014). *24/7: Late Capitalism and the Ends of Sleep*, London: Verso.
4 Gabel, *False Consciousness*, p. 121.

5 L. Wing (1975). 'Mentally retarded children in Camberwell (London)', in H. Hafner (ed.), *Estimating Needs for Mental Health Care*. Berlin: Springer. L. Wing and J. Gould (1979). 'Severe impairments of social interaction aud associated abnormalities in children: epidemiology and classification', *Journal of Autism and Childhood Schizophrenia* 9, 11–29.

6 F. Guattari (1995). *Chaosophy*. Cambridge, MA: MIT Press, p. 234.

7 D. Murray et al. (2005). 'Attention, monotropism, and the diagnostic criteria for autism', *Autism* 9(2), 139–56.

8 Douglas, *Purity and Danger*, p. 130.

9 R. Jordan and S. Powell (1995). *Understanding and Teaching Children with Autism*. New York: Wiley; M. Ives and N. Munro (2001). *Caring for a Child with Autism: A Practical Guide*. London: Jessica Kingsley.

10 Withington, *The Politics of Commonwealth*, p. 77.

11 Withington, p. 130.

12 Cited in Withington, p. 240.

13 S. Baron-Cohen (1991). 'Precursors to a theory of mind: understanding attention in others', in A. Whiten (ed.), *Natural Theories of Mind: Evolution, Development and Simulation of Everyday Mindreading*. Oxford: Blackwell.

14 M. Mauss (1924/1966). *The Gift*. Trans. Ian Cunnison. London: Cohen and West, p. 5.

15 W. Scott, *Essay on Drapery*, cited in Withington, *The Politics*, p. 140.

16 S. Baron-Cohen and S. Wheelwright (2004). 'The empathy quotient: an investigation of adults with Asperger syndrome or high functioning autism, and normal sex differences', *Journal of Autism and Developmental Disorders* 34(2), 163–75.

17 See for example S. Greenspan (2004). *The Greenspan Social Emotional Growth Chart: A Screening Questionnaire for Infants and Young Children*. New York: Pearson.

18 U. Frevert (2011). *Emotions in History – Lost and Found*. Budapest: Central European University Press.

19 A. Smith (1759/2002). *A Theory of Moral Sentiments*. Cambridge: Cambridge University Press, p. 180.

20 D. Hume (1751/1948). *An Enquiry concerning the Principles of Morals*, in H.Aitken (ed.), *Hume: Moral and Political Philosophy*. London: Macmillan. p. 217.

21 T. Browne (1642/1969). *Religio Medici*. Littlehampton: Everyman's Library, p. 81.

22 M. Nussbaum (2003). *Upheavals of Thought: The Intelligence of Emotions*. Cambridge: Cambridge University Press.

23 S. Baron-Cohen (2012). *Zero Degrees of Empathy: A New Understanding of Cruelty and Kindness*. London: Penguin.

24 D. Batson (2009). 'These things called empathy: eight related but distinct phenomena', in J. Decety and W. Ickes (eds), *The Social Neuroscience of Empathy*. Cambridge, MA: MIT Press.

25 See for example C. Pedwell (2014). *Affective Relations: The Transnational Politics of Empathy*. London: Macmillan.

26 J. Panksepp and G. Lahvis (2011). 'Rodent empathy and affective neuroscience', *Neuroscience and Biobehavioral Reviews* 35, 1864–1875.

27 S. Baron-Cohen (2009). 'Autism: the empathizing–systemizing (E–S) theory', in M. Miller and A. Kingstone (eds), *The Year in Cognitive Neuroscience*. New York: The New York Academy of Sciences, pp. 68–80.

28 A. Senju et al. (2007). 'Absence of contagious yawning in children with autism spectrum disorder', *Biology Letters* 3, 706–708; F. Giganti and Z. Esposito (2009) 'Contagious and spontaneous yawning in autistic and typically developing children', *Current Psychology Letters* 25, 1–11.

29 M. Helt et al. (2010). 'Contagious yawning in autistic and typical development', *Child Development* 81(5).

30 C. Morrison (2007). Paper given at British Association Festival of Science, York, September.

31 M. Campbell and F. de Waal, 'Ingroup-outgroup bias in contagious yawning by chimpanzees supports link to empathy', *PloS One* 6(4): e18283. doi: 10.1371/journal. pone.001828. Retrieved 6 December 2013.

32 Withington, *The Politics of Commonwealth*, p. 210.

33 See J. Tosh (1999). *A Man's Place: Masculinity and the Middle-Class Home in Victorian England.* New Haven, CT: Yale University Press. M. Poovey (1988). *Uneven Developments: The Ideological Work of Gender in Mid-Victorian England.* Chicago: University of Chicago Press.

34 D. Cullen (1994). 'Feminism, management and self-actualization', *Gender, Work and Orgnization* 1(3).

35 See also M. Waltz (2008). 'Autism = death: the social and medical impact of a catastrophic medical model of autistic spectrum disorders', *Popular Narrative Media* 1(1), 13–24. E-print.

36 C. Pedwell (2012). 'Affective (self-) transformations: empathy, neoliberalism and international development', *Feminist Theory* 13(2), 163–79.

37 R. Holmes (1965). 'Freud, Piaget and democratic leadership,' *British Journal of Sociology* 16, p. 123.

38 See Alderson (2013). *Childhoods Real and Imagined*; Alderson and Goodey (1995). 'Research with disabled children: how useful is child-centred ethics?' *Children and Society*, 12.

10 Conclusion

At the end of a wide-ranging canvas like this the reader might expect some grand predictions. And that is probably what you would get if you asked a practitioner in biogenetic research: a future free from learning disabilities, as well as from the people with them. Given their wide-ranging and ill-defined scope, this seems unlikely. Moreover, the prospect is hindered by fellow practitioners in the field of medicine and biotechnology who rescue increasingly early-term foetuses with disabilities more significant than those eliminated by pre-natal testing. We have seen the future and it does not work. At least, it is not perfection or cyborgs; it is an ordinary mess, just like the present and the past.

If you have got this far, the kind of grand prediction you are more likely to expect and want is a blueprint for liberation. It would not be difficult. For adults independence in the community, friendships, employment; for children a desegregated education system; for foetuses truly 'informed' consent, the main component of which would be monitoring for inclusion phobia among the informers, and a single date for permissible termination and permissible rescue; for the rest of us, an ordinary life that is only ordinary as long as people with learning difficulties are in it.

Their exclusion and their very existence as a separate category of human being, as we have seen, are the cornerstone of the disordered hierarchies and crises of differentiation that constantly disrupt the ingroup of the normally intelligent. For young people, ordinary lives would mean the abolition not only of segregated schools but also of selective and private ones. In universities, it would mean opening the life of enquiry to those without prior qualifications or not seeking a degree. It would mean a single accreditation system, for those skills where accreditation seems necessary, covering the apprentice hairdresser along with student of medicine or astrophysics. People with learning difficulties, of whatever level of severity, would be around in higher education since they have the same aspiration to enquire and learn as anyone else. There are pockets of existing practice that show all this is feasible, both for children and for adults, and in the UK they are spreading. However, they are also piecemeal and small. What are the prospects for overall change?

Change in the form of liberation is sometimes presented in a utopian format. One school of thought sees the very existence of services and expert professions as being the problem. All that has to be achieved is a society where people with learning difficulties and other 'vulnerable' people are supported organically, by their local community.[1] Indeed, it was from this school of thought that the very principles of person-centred planning arose, among advocates involved in the closure of institutions who sought to answer the question 'What are these people actually going to be doing?' and from thence to inclusive education.[2] An appropriate study of historical context in the distant past might find that organic community support was the norm at the start of human cultures, and we might certainly encourage it as a vision for the future. People are daily confronted with the fact that services *per se* are what prevents ordinary lives and inclusion in mainstream social institutions, and that expert assessment creates identity through 'clienthood' and in so doing seems to exist only to provide jobs for the relevant professionals and large voluntary organizations.

However, while the separate existence of expert and service professions is something that needs to be dealt with, it is not the first thing. It is counterproductive to wishfully think that one can *bypass* the era of services as of now, or to avoid engaging with existing providers and policy makers: that the medical utopia of a world without learning disability can be diverted by the social utopia, at least here and now, of a world without services. The neighbourhood politics slogan, The Revolution Starts Here, may be valid, and one should certainly behave as if that were the case. But how does revolution, particularly if it is local, penetrate whole systems? 'Don't go near government' may be a solution for some individuals in local situations, but not to the more fundamental problem of inclusion phobia as a whole.

Failure to recognize the ongoing historically contingent character of learning disability and of 'vulnerable people' generally means that the more permanent-looking structures of discrimination can always be renewed. In this book I have drawn links between present-day learning disability and some of the historical manifestations of inclusion phobia that bear no connection to it. Those links between the wildly differing targets of inclusion phobia across history may be tenuous. But what it also suggests is that the individuals *currently* labelled by learning disability may have only a very tenuous link *with each other*. What if their extreme outgroup status, being determined by an ingroup whose socio-historical profile is clearly arbitrary, is the only thing that unites and defines them?

Making blueprints for an imagined society in which the more fundamental pathology of inclusion phobia will not exist cannot be the primary task. It *does* exist. Our heads must start from somewhere other than utopia. The task is a political one. This is not to say that the phobia is the driver at policy levels – those of national government, remote from daily practice, or even of local government and administration. Here, among those with overall responsibility for the system, the driver is indifference and cowardice.

Indifference results from the fact that, for administrators, these people do not matter. They are just not important enough. The UK Department of Education can order the minutest changes to education (exam qualifications, for example) at the drop of a hat, but it will not order schools to deal with the refusal to enact its own inclusion policy or block the legal loopholes to it. Government can order the closure of all residential assessment and treatment centres but admit only puzzlement when repeated committees report that they continue to flourish, along with the abuse they generate. And because in its modern manifestation inclusion phobia classifies children as idiots too, if temporary ones, government is incapable of drawing the dots from educational segregation in childhood to the 'challenging behaviour' of adults in residential placements, who would be less likely to challenge others if they had grown up knowing that they were part of the same ordinary life and valued accordingly.

Cowardice consists in failure to stand up to the intelligence society's narcissistic bullying, which occurs at a personal level. People who do not matter, as a general category, exist in inverse correlation with the strength and ability of the rest of us to face down the people whose very job it is to ensure that they do not matter. Where the phobia and insanity are endemic is in the daily life of systems and institutions, and in the behaviour of individuals with power. Even here, it is possible to do something. At the private nursery school where Jonny (from Chapter 2) started his education, there was a unanimous strike threat when the head wanted him out. He stayed.

The above analysis, however, also overlooks the good intentions and actual effectiveness of people with responsibility for making the policy of person-centred planning work in practice, and as intended, i.e. emanating from the aspirations of individuals rather than from the external assessments of people observing them. That is another reason why the problem cannot be reduced to a battle between services and experts on the one hand and lay people on the other. Some small administrative steps in themselves can have a revolutionary impact. For a century and a half, coinciding with the rise of psychology as a formal discipline and the belated invasion of the field by medical science, the individual personality has been fragmented by assessment into a number of separate identities – imposed typically by social work, education and health, though these too are broken down into innumerable sub-specialisms – whose very conceptual basis mirrors the delusional nature of inclusion phobia. They see who the person is through the distorting lens of morbid rationalism, through the legacy of the long-stay institutions and the conceptual framework they generated, which steals the personal identities of people with learning difficulties from them at birth and determines who they will be. Person-centred planning, with its basis in single service plans, thus has the potential to shift one of the long-term tectonic plates of abuse.

The fact that we may be able to see in some modest policy steps a revolutionary significance for the future is why we end here not in a grand scheme but scrabbling around in the minutiae of daily practice. In the long perspective such steps may seem gradualist, but they are gradualist in a direction that does not compromise the principle and the primary challenge, that of combating inclusion phobia. If we are going to start from where we currently are, they are the footholds that do not allow for going backwards.

This does not stop us from thinking on a grander scale too. National and local government can recognize inclusion phobia by name and make it the foundation stone of social policy. They can divert funding from cognitive and behavioural genetics to university psychology and social science departments that will research the phobia's malign presence in practice and in everyday life, and will devise ways of eliminating it. Inclusion phobia should be recognized as a psychiatric disorder in its own right; the next edition of psychiatry's *Diagnostic and Statistical Manual* can itemize it expressly, in its appropriate place alongside specific phobia. As a general feature of modern societies, it needs to be combated not only in terms of systems but equally in the everyday behaviour of individuals who suffer from it and who nevertheless often have great power over people's lives.

Persuading, educating, campaigning, changing the law, getting it to work when it has changed, providing clear proof that inclusion works – these have already had an influence in discrete ways and are not to be discouraged. But the evidence is also that on their own they will fail to make the overall impact that is needed. And that is because they are about the wrong thing. Inclusion is not a good idea that needs to be promoted, it is the state of nature. Only in an entirely unnatural situation is inclusion something that has to be asked for or fought for. If the disorder lies in the ingroup, that is logically where the policy focus has to be.

Notes

1 J. McKnight (1995). *The Careless Society: Community and Its Counterfeits.* New York: Basic Books; S. Thomas and W. Wolfensberger (1999). 'An overview of social role valorization', in R. Flynn and R. Lemay (eds), *A Quarter Century of Normalization and Social Role Valorization: Evolution and Impact.* Ottawa: University of Ottawa Press.
2 C. O'Brien and J. O'Brien (2002). 'The origins of person-centered planning: a community of practice perspective', in S. Holburn and P. Vietze (eds), *Research and Practice in Person-Centered Planning.* Baltimore, MD: Brookes.

References

J. Able (2008–9). *Cold Stone Floors and Carbolic Soap.* www.richmond.gov.uk/our_tim es_newsletter_march_09.pdf and www.richmond.gov.uk/our_times_autumn_2008. pdf. Retrieved 14 April 2014.

Advertisement for Brookdale Care (byline, 'Brookdale: exclusively autism') in *Community Care*, 7 October 2010.

G. Agamben (1998). *Homo Sacer: Sovereign Power and Bare Life.* Stanford, CA: Stanford University Press.

Albertus Magnus. *Ethica* I.47, in *Works Online.* www.albertusmagnus.uwaterloo.ca

P. Alderson (2013). *Childhoods Real and Imagined.* Abingdon: Routledge.

P. Alderson and C. Goodey (1995). 'Research with disabled children: how useful is child-centred ethics?' *Children and Society* 10(2), 106–116.

P. Alderson and C. Goodey (1999). *Enabling Education: Experiences in Special and Ordinary Schools.* London: Falmer.

G. Aly, P. Chroust and C. Pross (1994). *Cleansing the Fatherland: Nazi Medicine and Racial Hygiene*, Baltimore, MD: Johns Hopkins University Press.

American Psychiatric Association (2013). *Diagnostic and Statistical Manual of Mental Disorders.* 5th edn, Arlington VA: American Psychiatric Publishing.

P. W. Anderson (1997). 'Is measurement itself an emergent property?' *Complexity* 3(1), 14–16.

C. Ando (2000). *Imperial Ideology and Provincial Loyalty in the Roman Empire.* Los Angeles: University of California Press.

P. Aries (1962). *Centuries of Childhood.* New York: Vintage.

W. H. Auden (1976). 'Luther', in *Collected Poems* (ed. E. Mendelson). London: Faber.

P. Balasundaram (2005). *Sunny's Story.* Delhi: ISPCK.

O. Barden (2012). 'Facebook as a catalyst for critical literacy learning by dyslexic sixth-form students', *Literacy* 46(3), 123–132.

S. Baron-Cohen (1991). 'Precursors to a theory of mind: understanding attention in others', in A. Whiten (ed.), *Natural Theories of Mind: Evolution, Development and Simulation of Everyday Mindreading.* Oxford: Blackwell.

S. Baron-Cohen (2009). 'Autism: the empathizing–systemizing (E-S) theory', in M. Miller and A. Kingstone (eds), *The Year in Cognitive Neuroscience.* New York: The New York Academy of Sciences, 68–80.

S. Baron-Cohen (2012). *Zero Degrees of Empathy: A New Understanding of Cruelty and Kindness.* London: Penguin.

S. Baron-Cohen and S. Wheelwright (2004). 'The empathy quotient: an investigation of adults with Asperger syndrome or high functioning autism, and normal sex differences'. *Journal of Autism and Developmental Disorders* 34(2), 2004, 163–175.

S. Baron-Cohen, A. Leslie and U. Frith (1985). 'Does the autistic child have a theory of mind?' *Cognition* 21, 37–46.

P. Bartlett and D. Wright (1999). 'Community care and its antecedents', in P. Bartlett and D. Wright, *Outside the Walls of the Asylum: The History of Care in the Community 1750–2000*. London: Athlone.

D. Batson (2009). 'These things called empathy: eight related but distinct phenomena', in J. Decety and W. Ickes (eds), *The Social Neuroscience of Empathy*. Cambridge MA: MIT Press.

M. Bayat (2015). 'The stories of "snake children": the killing and abuse of children with developmental disabilities in West Africa', *Journal of Intellectual Disability Research* 59(1), 1–10.

C. Bennett, A. Baird, M. Miller and G. Wolford (2010). 'Neural correlates of inter-species perspective taking in the post-mortem Atlantic Salmon: an argument for proper multiple comparisons correction', *Journal of Serendipitous and Unexpected Results* 1(1), 1–5.

G. Berrios and I. Markova (2002). 'Conceptual issues', in H. D'haenen, J. Den Boer and P. Willner (eds), *Biological Psychiatry*, New York: Wiley.

A. Binet (1905). 'Méthodes nouvelles pour le diagnostic du niveau intellectuel des anormaux,' *L'année psychologique*, 11, 191–244.

C. Blacker (1947). *Problem Families: Five Inquiries*. London: Eugenics Society.

A. Boggis (2011). 'Deafening silences: researching with inarticulate children', *Disability Studies Quarterly*, 31(4), 1–7.

T. (Tim) Booth (1978). 'From normal baby to handicapped child', *Sociology* 12, 203–221.

T. (Tim) Booth and W. Booth (1996). 'Sounds of silence: narrative research with inarticulate subjects', *Disability and Society* 11(1), 55–69.

T. (Tony) Booth and M. Ainscow (2002). *Index for Inclusion: Developing Learning and Participation in Schools*. Bristol: CSIE.

N. Bostrom and A. Sandberg (2009). 'Cognitive enhancement: methods, ethics, regulatory enhancements', *Science and Engineering Ethics* 15, 311–341.

N. Bostrom (2008). 'Why I want to be a posthuman when I grow up', in B. Gordijn and R. Chadwick (eds), *Medical Enhancement and Postumanity*. Berlin: Springer.

B. Bradley (1989). *Visions of Infancy: Critical Introduction to Child Psychology*. Cambridge: Polity.

M. Braine and D. O'Brien (eds) (1998). *Mental Logic*. Mahwah, NJ: Lawrence Erlbaum.

T. Browne (1642/1969). *Religio Medici*. Littlehampton: Everyman's Library.

J. Bruner and C. Goodman (1947). 'Value and need as organizing factors in perception', *Journal of Abnormal and Social Psychology*, 42, 33–34.

H. Brunius (2007). *Better for All the World: The Secret History of Forced Sterilization and America's Quest for Racial Purity*. New York: Vintage.

J. Bunyan (1674). *Reprobation Asserted*. London: G.L.

K. Burke (1969). *A Grammar of Motives*. Berkeley: University of California Press.

M. Burleigh (1994). *Death and Deliverance: Euthanasia in Germany 1900–1945*. Cambridge: Cambridge University Press.

R. Burton (1621/1973). *The Anatomy of Melancholy*. Littlehampton: Everyman's University Library.

K. Button, J. Ioannidis, C. Mosryk, B. Nosek, J. Flint, E. Robinson and M. Munafò (2013). 'Power failure: why small sample size undermines the reliability of neuroscience', *Nature Reviews Neuroscience*, 14(5), 365–376.

M. Campbell and F. de Waal (2013). 'Ingroup-outgroup bias in contagious yawning by chimpanzees supports link to empathy', *PloS One* 6(4): e18283. doi: 10.1371/journal. pone.001828. Retrieved 6 December 2013.

G. Canguilhem (1989). *The Normal and the Pathological*. New York: Zone.

P. Chance (1974). '"After you hit a child, you can't just get up and leave him; you are hooked to that kid". A conversation with Ivor Lovaas about self-mutilating children and how their parents make it worse', *Psychology Today* 7(8), 76–84.

L. Chapman (1967). 'Illusory correlation in observational report,' *Journal of Verbal Learning and Verbal Behaviour* 6(1), 151–155.

I. Chen (2013). 'Hidden depths', *New Scientist* 220, 19 October.

P. Churchland (1986). *Neurophilosophy: Toward a Unified Science of the Mind-Brain*. Cambridge, MA: MIT Press.

J. Clapton (2009). *A Transformatory Ethic of Inclusion*. Rotterdam: Sense.

R. Collingwood (2005). *The Idea of History*. Revised edn. Oxford: Oxford University Press.

Columbia University Medical Centre, 'Children with autism have extra synapses in brain', http://newsroom.cumc.columbia.edu/blog/2014/08/21/children-autism-extra-synap ses-brain/. Retrieved 2 December 2014.

M. Cooper (2012). *I'd Like to Know Why*. Ashill: Clover Press.

J. Crary (2014). *24/7: Late Capitalism and the Ends of Sleep*. London: Verso.

D. Cullen (1994). 'Feminism, management and self-actualisation', *Gender, Work and Orgnization* 1(3), 127–137.

K. Danziger (1990). *Constructing the Subject: Historical Origins of Psychological Research*. Cambridge: Cambridge University Press.

K. Danziger (1997). *Naming the Mind: How Psychology Found its Language*. London: Sage.

F. Darwin (1887). *The Life and Letters of Charles Darwin, Including an Autobiographical Chapter*. London: John Murray.

J. Das, J. Naglieri and J. Kirby (1994). *Assessment of Cognitive Processes*. Needham Heights, MA: Allyn & Bacon.

J. Davenport, 'Warning as number of witchcraft child abuse cases rise in London', *London Evening Standard*, 9 October 2014.

R. Dawkins (1989). *The Extended Phenotype*. Oxford: Oxford University Press.

A. Daye (1586/1635). *The Second Part of the English Secretorie*. London: Stansby.

R. Descartes (1983). *Oeuvres*. Paris: Vrin.

A. Desmond and J. Moore (1991). *Darwin*. London: Michael Joseph.

D. Detterman. *Human Intelligence: Historical Influences, Current Controversies, Teaching Resources*, at http://intelltheory.com/detterman.shtml. Retrieved 28 November 2014.

M. Donaldson (1978). *Children's Minds*. London: Fontana.

M. Douglas (1966). *Purity and Danger: An Analysis of Concepts of Pollution and Taboo*. London: Routledge.

R. Dunbar (2004). 'Gossip in evolutionary perspective', *Review of General Psychology* 8(2), 100–110.

J. Dupré (2012). *Processes of Life: Essays in the Philosophy of Biology*. Oxford: Oxford University Press.

T. Eagleton (2000). *The Idea of Culture*. Oxford: Blackwell.

Easter Seals Disability Services, Chicago (2014). http://blog.easterseals.com/are-paren ts-of-children-with-autism-heroes. Retrieved 27 December 2014.

B. Evans (2013). 'How autism became autism: the radical transformation of a central concept of child development in Britain', *History of the Human Sciences* 26(3), 3–31.

M. Falvey, M. Forest, J. Pearpoint and R. Rosenberg (1997). *All My Life's a Circle. Using the Tools: Circles, Maps and Paths*. Toronto: Inclusion Press.

R. Fenn (1995). *The Persistence of Purgatory*. Cambridge: Cambridge University Press.

P. Ferguson (1994). *Abandoned to their Fate: Social Policy and Practice toward Severely Retarded People in America, 1820–1920*. Philadelphia: Temple University Press.

R. Feuerstein (1990). 'The theory of structural modifiability', in B. Presseisen (ed.), *Learning and Thinking Styles: Classroom Interaction*. Washington, DC: National Education Associations.

S. Firestein (2012). *Ignorance: How It Drives Science*. Oxford: Oxford University Press.

B. Firestone (2007). *Autism Heroes: Portraits of Families Meeting the Challenge*. London: Jessica Kingsley.

P. Fisher and D. Goodley (2007). 'The linear medical model of disability: mothers of disabled babies resist', *Sociology of Health and Illness* 29(1), 66–81.

M. Flynn (2012). *Serious Case Review: Winterbourne View Hospital*. South Gloucestershire Council.

D. Freeman, P. Garety, E. Kuipers, D. Fowler and P. Bebbington (2002). 'A cognitive model of persecutory delusions', *British Journal of Clinical Psychology* 41, 331–347.

U. Frevert (2011). *Emotions in History: Lost and Found*. Budapest: Central European University Press.

C. Frith (2007). *Making Up the Mind: How the Brain Creates Our Mental World*. Oxford: Blackwell.

U. Frith (1989). *Autism: Explaining the Enigma*. Oxford: Blackwell.

U. Frith (1992). *Autism and Asperger Syndrome*. Cambridge: Cambridge University Press.

J. Gabel (1975). *False Consciousness: An Essay on Reification*. Oxford: Blackwell.

J. Gabel (1997). *Ideologies*. New Brunswick, NJ: Transaction.

F. Galton (1869). *Hereditary Genius: An Inquiry into Its Laws and Consequences*. London: Macmillan.

H. Gardner (2008). 'Wrestling with Jean Piaget, my paragon'. *The World Question Center*, www.edge.org/q2011/q11_index.html. Retrieved 11 September 2014.

H. Gardner (2011). *Frames of Mind: The Theory of Multiple Intelligences*. New York: Basic Books.

K. Gergen (1985). 'The social constructionist movement in modern psychology', *American Psychologist* 40, 266–375.

F. Giganti and Z. Esposito (2009). 'Contagious and spontaneous yawning in autistic and typically developing children', *Current Psychology Letters* 25, 1–11.

T. Gineste (1981). *Victor de l'Aveyron: dernier enfant sauvage, premier enfant fou*. Paris: Sycomore.

R. Girard (1986). *The Scapegoat*. Translated by Y. Freccero. Baltimore, MD: Johns Hopkins University Press.

E. Goffman (1961). *Asylums: Essays on the Social Situation of Mental Patients and Other Inmates*. New York: Doubleday.

J. Goldenberg (2001). 'I am not an animal: mortality salience, disgust, and the denial of human creatureliness', *Journal of Experimental Psychology* 130(3), 427–435.

B. Goode (2011). *The Goode Life: Memoirs of Disability Rights Activist Barb Goode*. Vancouver: Spectrum.

C. Goodey (1997). 'Genes that are all in the mind', *New Scientist*, 7 June.

C. Goodey (2011). *A History of Intelligence and 'Intellectual Disability': The Shaping of Psychology in Early Modern Europe*. Farnham: Ashgate.

C. Goodey and M. Rose (2013). 'Mental states, bodily dispositions and table manners: a guide to reading "intellectual" disability from Homer to late Antiquity', in C. Laes, C. Goodey and M. Rose (eds), *Disabilities in Roman Antiquity: Disparate Bodies, a Capite ad Calcem*. Leiden: Brill.

C. Goodey and T. Stainton (2001). 'Intellectual disability and the myth of the changeling myth', *Journal for the History of the Behavioural Sciences* 37(3), 223–240.

D. Goodley (2001). "Learning difficulties", the social model of disability and impairment: challenging epistemologies', *Disability and Society* 16(2), 207–231.

L. Gottfredson (1997). 'Mainstream science on intelligence: an editorial with 52 signatories, history, and bibliography', *Intelligence* 24(1), 13–23.

S. Gould (1996). *The Mismeasure of Man*. New York: Norton.

I. Green (1996). *The Christian's ABC: Catechisms and Catechizing in England c.1530–1740*. Oxford: Clarendon Press.

S. Greenspan (2004). *The Greenspan Social Emotional Growth Chart: A Screening Questionnaire for Infants and Young Children*. New York: Pearson.

P. Griffiths (2012). 'Dancing in the dark: evolutionary psychology and the argument from design', in S. Scher and F. Rauscher (eds), *Evolutionary Psychology: Alternative Approaches*. New York: Springer.

F. Guattari (1995). *Chaosophy*. Cambridge, MA: MIT Press.

J. Guilford (1988). 'Some changes in the structure of intellect model', *Educational and Psychological Measurement, 48*, 1–4.

J. Guilford (1967). *The Nature of Human Intelligence*. New York: McGraw-Hill.

I. Hacking (2004a). 'Between Michel Foucault and Erving Goffman: between discourse in the abstract and face-to-face interaction', *Economy and Society* 33(3), 277–302.

I. Hacking (2004b). *Historical Ontology*. Cambridge, MA: Harvard University Press.

I. Hacking (2006a). 'Making up people', *London Review of Books* 28(16), 23–26.

I. Hacking, (2006b). 'What is Tom saying to Maureen?' *London Review of Books* 28(9), 3–7.

L. Harris (2006). 'Dehumanizing the lowest of the low: neuroimaging responses to extreme outgroups', *Psychological Science* 17, 847–853.

L. Haynes, O. Service, B. Goldacre and D. Torgerson (2012). *Test, Learn, Adapt: Developing Public Policy with Randomised Control Trials*. London: Cabinet Office Behavioural Insights Team.

D. Healy (1997). *The Antidepressant Era*. Cambridge, MA: Harvard University Press.

M. Helt, I. Eigsti, P. Snyder and D. Fein (2010). 'Contagious yawning in autistic and typical development', *Child Development* 81(5), 1620–1631.

N. Hervey (1986). 'Advocacy or folly: the Alleged Lunatics' Friend Society, 1845–1863', *Medical History* 30, 245–275.

E. Hillesum (2014). *The Complete Works 1941–43*, eds K. Smelik and M. Coetsier. Aachen: Shaker.

R. Holmes (1965). 'Freud, Piaget and democratic leadership', *British Journal of Sociology* 16, 123–139.

R. Houston and U. Frith (2000). *Autism in History: The Case of Hugh Blair of Borgue*. Oxford: Blackwell.

J. Huarte (1594/1969). *The Examination of Men's Wits*. Amsterdam: Da Capo Press.

M. Huerta, S. Bishop, A. Duncan, V. Hus and C. Lord (2012). 'Application of DSM-5 criteria for autism spectrum disorder to three samples of children with DSM-IV diagnoses of pervasive developmental disorders', *American Journal of Psychiatry* 169(10), 1056–1064.

B. Hughes and K. Patterson (1997). 'The social model of disability and the disappearing body: towards a sociology of impairment', *Disability and Society* 12(3), 325–340.

R. Hughes, M. Redley and M. Ring (2011). 'Friendship and adults with profound intellectual and multiple disabilities and English disability policy', *Journal of Policy and Practice in Intellectual Disabilities* 8(3), 197–206.

D. Hume (1751/1948). *An Enquiry Concerning the Principles of Morals*, in H. Aitken (ed.), *Hume: Moral and Political Philosophy*. London: Macmillan.

J. Ioannidis, E. Ntzani, T. Trikalinos and D. Contopoulos-Ioannidis (2001). 'Replication validity of genetic association studies', *Nature Genetics* 29, 306–309.

P. Irwing and R. Lynn (2005). 'Sex differences in means and variability on the Progressive Matrices in university students: a meta-analysis', *British Journal of Psychology* 96, 505–524.

M. Ives and N. Munro (2001). *Caring for a Child with Autism: A Practical Guide*. London: Jessica Kingsley.

M. Jackson (2000). *The Borderland of Imbecility: Medicine, Society and the Fabrication of the Feeble Mind in Later Victorian and Edwardian England*. Manchester: Manchester University Press.

N. Ji, G. Capone and W. Kaufmann (2011). 'Autism spectrum disorder in Down syndrome: cluster analysis of aberrant behaviour checklist data supports diagnosis', *Journal of Intellectual Disability Research* 55(11), 1064–1077.

L. Jordan and C. Goodey (1996). *Human Rights and School Change*. Bristol: CSIE.

R. Jordan and S. Powell (1995). *Understanding and Teaching Children with Autism*. New York: Wiley.

J. Joseph and N. Wetzel (2013). 'Ernst Rüdin: Hitler's racial hygiene mastermind', *Journal for the History of Biology* 46(1), 1–30.

I. Kant (1791/1960). *Religion Within the Limits of Reason Alone*, trs T. Greene and H. Hudson. New York: Harper & Row.

A. Karmiloff-Smith (2006). 'The tortuous route from genes to behaviour: a neuroconstructivist approach', *Cognitive, Affective, and Behavioral Neuroscience* 6(1), 9–17.

A. Karmiloff-Smith (2010). 'Neuroimaging of the developing brain: taking "developing" seriously', *Human Brain Mapping* 31(6), 934–941.

R. Keller (2007). *Colonial Madness: Psychiatry in French North Africa*. Chicago: University of Chicago Press.

T. Kelley (1929). *Scientific Method*. Ohio: Ohio State University Press.

D. Kirby (2000). 'The new eugenics in cinema: genetic determinism and gene therapy in *Gattaca*', *Science Fiction Studies* 27(2), 193–215.

P. Kitcher (1989). 'Explanatory unification and the causal structure of the world', in P. Kitcher and W. Salmon (eds), *Scientific Explanation*. Minneapolis: University of Minnesota Press.

K. Kosik (1976). *Dialectics of the Concrete: A Study of Problems of Man and World*. Dordrecht: Reidel.

A. Krosch and D. Amodio (2014). 'Economic scarcity alters the perception of race', *Proceedings of the National Academy of Sciences* 111(45), 9079–9084.

C. Kudlick (2003). 'Disability history: why we need another other', *American Historical Review* 108(3), 763–793.

J. Leask, A. Leask and N. Silove (2005). 'Evidence for autism in folklore?' *Archives of Disease in Childhood* 90(3), 271.

M. Leboyer, F. Bellivier, M. Nosten-Bertrrand, R. Jouvent, D. Pauls and J. Mallet (1998). 'Psychiatric genetics: search for phenotypes', *Trends in Neurosciences* 21(3), 102–105.

J. Locke (1689/1975). *An Essay Concerning Human Understanding*. Oxford: Clarendon Press.

J. Locke (1689/1998). *Two Treatises of Government*. Cambridge: Cambridge University Press.

R. Lynn (2002). 'Skin color and intelligence in African Americans,' *Population and Environment* 23(4), 365–375.

P. McDonagh (2007). 'Autism and modernism: a genealogical exploration', in M. Osteen (ed.), *Autism and Representation*. Abingdon: Routledge.

P. McDonagh (2008). *Idiocy: A Cultural History*. Liverpool: Liverpool University Press.

J. McDonald (2013). 'Making the world safe for eugenics: the eugenicist Harry H. Laughlin's encounters with American internationalism', *Journal of the Gilded Age and Progressive Era* 12(3), 379–411.

J. McKnight (1995). *The Careless Society: Community and Its Counterfeits*. New York: Basic Books.

M. Mauss (1924/1966). *The Gift*. Translated by Ian Cunnison. London: Cohen and West.

M. Mauss (1972). *A General Theory of Magic*. Translated by Robert Brain. London: Routledge.

J. Meiland (1965). *Skepticism and Historical Knowledge*. New York: Random House.

I. Metzler (2016). *Fools and Idiots? Intellectual Disability in the Middle Ages*. Manchester: Manchester University Press.

J. Michell (1999). *Measurement in Psychology: A Critical History of a Methodological Concept*. Cambridge: Cambridge University Press.

M. Miles (2010). *The Chuas of Sha Daulah at Gujrat, Pakistan: Evidence, Historical Background and Development, with Bibliography, 1839–2009*. Stockholm: Independent Living Institute.

D. Mitchell with S. Snyder (2015). *The Biopolitics of Disability: Neoliberalism, Ablenationalism, and Peripheral Embodiment*. Ann Arbor: University of Michigan Press.

P. Monaghan and T. Birkhead (2013). 'Variety: the spice of life sciences', *Times Higher Education Supplement*, 27 June.

R. Moore (2007). *The Formation of a Persecutory Society: Authority and Deviance in Western Europe 950–1250*. Oxford: Blackwell.

R. Moore (2012). *The War on Heresy: Faith and Power in Medieval Europe*. London: Profile Books.

C. Morrison (2007). 'Contagious yawning', Paper given at British Association Festival of Science, York, September. Cited in J. Collingwood, 'Researchers tackle the mystery of yawning', http://psychcentral.com/lib/

A. Murray (1978). *Reason and Society in the Middle Ages*. Oxford: Oxford University Press.

D. Murray, M. Lesser and W. Lawson (2005). 'Attention, monotropism, and the diagnostic criteria for autism', *Autism* 9(2), 139–156.

M. Nadesan (2005). *Constructing Autism: Unravelling the 'Truth' and Understanding the Social*. London: Routledge.

C. Navarrete and D. Fessler (2006). 'Disease avoidance and ethnocentrism: the effects of disease vulnerability and disgust sensitivity on intergroup attitudes', *Evolution and Human Behavior* 27(4), 270–282.

C. Neely (2004). *Distracted Subjects: Madness and Gender in Shakespeare and Early Modern Culture*. Ithaca, NY: Cornell University Press.

U. Neisser (1967). *Cognitive Psychology*. New York: Appleton-Century-Crofts.

U. Neisser, G. Boodoo, T. Bouchard, A. Boykin, N. Brody, S. Ceci, D. Halpern, J. Loehlin, R. Perloff, R. Sternberg and S. Urbina (1996). 'Intelligence: knowns and unknowns', *American Psychologist* 51(2), 77.

C. Nightingale (2012). *Segregation: A Global History of Divided Cities*. Chicago: University of Chicago Press.

R. Nisbett (2013). 'Schooling makes you smarter: what teachers need to know about IQ', *American Educator* Spring, 10–39.

R. Nisbett, J. Aronson, C. Blair, W. Dickens, J. Flynn, D. Halpern and E. Turkheimer (2012). 'Intelligence: new findings and theoretical developments', *American Psychologist* 67(2), 130–160.

M. Nussbaum (2003). *Upheavals of Thought: The Intelligence of Emotions*. Cambridge: Cambridge University Press.

M. Nussbaum (2007). *Frontiers of Justice: Disability, Nationality, Species Membership*. Cambridge, MA: Harvard University Press.

G. O'Brien (2013). *Framing the Moron: The Social Construction of Feeble-Mindedness in the American Eugenic Era*. Manchester: Manchester University Press.

C. O'Brien and J. O'Brien (2002). 'The origins of person-centered planning: a community of practice perspective', in S. Holburn and P. Vietze (eds), *Research and Practice in Person-Centered Planning*. Baltimore, MD: Brookes.

J. O'Brien and C. O'Brien (2006). *Implementing Person-Centred Planning: Voices of Experience*. Toronto: Inclusion Press.

B. Olatunji (2008). 'Core, animal reminder, and contamination disgust: three kinds of disgust with distinct personality, behavioral, physiological, and clinical correlates', *Journal of Research in Personality* 42(5), 1243–1259.

M. Oliver (1990). *The Politics of Disablement*. Basingstoke: Macmillan.

J. Panksepp and G. Lahvis (2011). 'Rodent empathy and affective neuroscience', *Neuroscience and Biobehavioral Reviews* 35, 1864–1875.

K. Patterson (1999). 'Disability studies and phenomenology: the carnal policies of everyday life', *Disability and Society* 14(5), 597–610.

C. Pedwell (2012). 'Affective (self-) transformations: empathy, neoliberalism and international development', *Feminist Theory* 13(2), 163–179.

C. Pedwell (2014). *Affective Relations: The Transnational Politics of Empathy*. London: Macmillan.

J. Piaget with B. Inhelder (1958). *The Growth of Logical Thinking from Childhood to Adolescence*. New York: Basic Books.

J. Piaget (1968). *Genetic Epistemology*. New York: Columbia University Press.

R. Plomin, J. DeFries, V. Knopik and J. Neiderhiser (2012). *Behavioral Genetics*. 6th edn. London and New York: Worth Publishers.

D. Plotz (2005). *The Genius Factory: The Curious History of the Nobel Prize Sperm Bank*. New York: Random House.

J. A. Plucker and A. Esping (eds) (2014). 'Human intelligence: historical influences, current controversies, teaching resources'. www.intelltheory.com. Retrieved 28 November 2014.

M. Poovey (1988). *Uneven Developments: The Ideological Work of Gender in Mid-Victorian England*. Chicago: University of Chicago Press.

T. Porter (1995). *Trust in Numbers: The Pursuit of Objectivity in Science and Public Life*. Princeton, NJ: Princeton University Press.

D. Premack and G. Woodruff (1978). 'Does the chimpanzee have a theory of mind?' *Behavioural and Brain Sciences* 1(4), 515–526.

J. Pring (2014). 'Inclusion is only right for some disabled children, says EHRC', *Disability News Service*, 24. www.disabilitynewsservice.com, retrieved 4 March 2014.

S. Rachman (2004). 'Fear of contamination', *Behavior Research and Therapy* 42(11), 1227–1255.

C. Rawcliffe (2006). *Leprosy in Medieval England*. Woodbridge, Suffolk: Boydell Press.

J. Rawls (1971). *A Theory of Justice*. Cambridge, MA: Harvard University Press.

K. Rodina (2006). 'Vygotsky's social constructionist view on disability: a methodology for inclusive education'. UCLA San Diego Laboratory of Comparative Human Cognition. www.lchc.ucsd.edu/MCA/paper. Retrieved 2 December 2014.

F. Rosen (2003). *Classical Utilitarianism from Hume to Mill*. London: Routledge.

M. Rothbart, S. Fulero, C. Jensen, J. Howard and P. Birrell (1978). 'From individual to group perspectives: availability heuristics in stereotype formation', *Journal of Experimental Social Psychology* 14, 237–255.

J.-J. Rousseau (1762/1979). *Emile, or On Education*. New York: Basic Books.

P. Rozin, L. Lowery, S. Imada and J. Haidt (1999). 'The CAD triad hypothesis: a mapping between three moral emotions (contempt, anger, disgust) and three moral codes (community, autonomy, divinity)', *Journal of Personality and Social Psychology* 76, 574–586.

A. Rutherford (2014). *Intelligence: Born Smart, Born Equal, Born Different*, aired 6 May, BBC Radio 4.

M. Rutter, L. Andersen-Wood, C. Beckett, D. Bredenkamp, J. Castle, C. Groothuis, J. Kreppner, L. Keaveney, C. Lord, T. O'Connor and the ERA Study Team (1999). 'Quasi-autistic patterns following severe early global privation', *Journal of Child Psychology and Psychiatry* 40(4), 537–549.

S. Sand (2009). *The Invention of the Jewish People*. London: Verso.

A. Sandberg and J. Savulescu (2011). 'The social and economic impacts of cognitive enhancement', in J. Savulescu, R. ter Meulen and G. Kahane (eds), *Enhancing Human Capacities*. New York: Wiley.

R. Schalock, S. Borthwick-Duffy, V. Bradley, W. Buntinx, D. Coulter, E. Craig, S. Gomez, Y. Lachapelle, R. Luckasson, A. Reeve, K. Shogren, M. Snell, S. Spreat, M. Tasse, J. Thompson, M. Verdugo-Alonso, M. Wehmeyer and M. Yeager (2007). 'The renaming of mental retardation: understanding the change to the term intellectual disability', *Intellectual and Developmental Disabilities* 45(2), 116–124.

R. Schalock, R. Luckasson and K. Shogren (2010). *Intellectual Disability: Definition, Classification and Systems of Support*. Washington, DC: AAIDD.

S. Scher and F. Rauscher (eds) (2012). *Evolutionary Psychology: Alternative Approaches*. New York: Springer.

R. Scruton (2011). 'Neurononsense and the soul', in J. Wentzel van Huyssteen and E. Wiebe (eds), *In Search of Self: Interdisciplinary Perspectives on Personhood*. Grand Rapids, MI: Eerdmans.

P. Sedgwick (1982). *PsychoPolitics*. New York: HarperCollins.

A. Senju, M. Maeda, Y. Kikuchi, T. Hasegawa, Y. Tojo and H. Osanai (2007). 'Absence of contagious yawning in children with autism spectrum disorder', *Biology Letters* 3, 706–708.

S. Seung (2012). *Connectome: How the Brain's Wiring Makes Us Who We Are*. New York: Houghton Mifflin.

T. Shakespeare (2006). *Disability Rights and Wrongs*. Abingdon: Routledge.

S. Shapin and S. Schaffer (1994). *A Social History of Truth: Civility and Science in Seventeenth-Century England*. Chicago: University of Chicago Press.

P. Shaw (2014). *Reading Dante: From Here to Eternity*. New York: Norton.

M. Shildrick (2009). *Dangerous Discourses of Disability, Subjectivity and Sexuality*. New York: Palgrave Macmillan.

C. Shulman and N. Bostrom (2014). 'Embryo selection for cognitive enhancement: curiosity or game-changer?' *Global Policy* 5(1), 85–92.

C. Silverman (2013). *Understanding Autism: Parents, Doctors, and the History of a Disorder*. Princeton, NJ: Princeton University Press.

M. Simpson (2007). 'From savage to citizen: education, colonialism and idiocy', *British Journal of Sociology of Education* 28(5), 561–574.

M. Simpson (2013). *Modernity and the Appearance of Idiocy: Intellectual Disability as a Regime of Truth*. Lampeter, Ceredigion: Edwin Mellen.

P. Singer (1994). *Rethinking Life and Death: The Collapse of Our Traditional Ethics*. New York: St. Martin's Press.

D. Skuse (2000). 'Behavioural phenotypes: what do they teach us?' *Archives of Disease in Childhood* 82, 222–225.

A. Smith (1759/2002). *A Theory of Moral Sentiments*. Cambridge: Cambridge University Press.

R. Smith (2007). *Being Human: Historical Knowledge and the Creation of Human Nature*. New York: Columbia University Press.

D. Smukler (2005). 'Unauthorized minds: how "theory of mind" theory misrepresents autism,' *Mental Retardation* 43, 11–24.

A. Solomon (2014). *Far from the Tree: Parents, Children and the Search for Identity*. New York: Vintage.

C. Spearman (1950). *Human Ability*. London: Macmillan.

P. Spikins (2009). 'Autism, the integrations of "difference" and the origins of modern human behaviour', *Cambridge Archaeological Journal* 19(2), 179–201.

T. Stainton (2001). 'Medieval charitable institutions and intellectual impairment c. 1066–1600', *Journal of Developmental Disabilities* 8(2), 19–29.

T. Stainton and H. Besser (1998). 'The positive impact of children with an intellectual disability on the family', *Journal of Intellectual and Developmental Disability* 23, 57–70.

R. Sternberg (1985). *Beyond IQ: A Triarchic Theory of Intelligence*. Cambridge: Cambridge University Press.

R. Sternberg (1997). *Successful Intelligence: How Practical and Creative Intelligence Determine Success in Life*. New York: Penguin Putnam.

R. Sternberg and D. Detterman (1986). *What Is Intelligence? Contemporary Viewpoints on Its Nature and Definition*. Norwood NJ: Ablex.

B. Stock (1983). *The Implications of Literacy: Written Language and Models of Interpretation in the Eleventh and Twelfth Centuries*. Princeton, NJ: Princeton University Press.

T. Suddendorf (2014). *The Gap: The Science of What Separates Us from Other Animals*. New York: Basic Books.

H. Tajfel (1981). *Human Groups and Social Categories*. Cambridge: Cambridge University Press.

M. Taylor (2014). *Speed Limits: Where Time Went and Why We Have So Little Left*. New Haven, CT: Yale University Press.

S. Taylor, J. Racino, J. Knoll and Z. Lutfiyya (1987). *The Nonrestrictive Environment: On Community Integration of Persons with the Most Severe Disabilities*. Syracuse, NY: Human Policy Press.

P. Teilhard de Chardin (1959). *The Phenomenon of Man*. London: Harper.

S. Thomas and W. Wolfensberger (1999). 'An overview of social role valorization', in R. Flynn and R. Lemay (eds), *A Quarter Century of Normalization and Social Role Valorization: Evolution and Impact*. Ottawa, Ontario: University of Ottawa Press.

M. Thomson (1998). *The Problem of Mental Deficiency: Eugenics, Democracy, and Social Policy in Britain c.1870–1959*. Oxford: Oxford University Press.

S. Timimi, N. Gardiner and B. MacCabe (2011). *The Myth of Autism*. London: Macmillan.

J. Tosh (1999). *A Man's Place: Masculinity and the Middle-Class Home in Victorian England*. New Haven, CT: Yale University Press.

J. Trent (1995). *Inventing the Feeble Mind: A History of Mental Retardation in the United States*. Berkeley: University of California Press.

J. Trent and S. Noll (2004). *Mental Retardation in America: A Historical Reader*. New York: New York University Press.

Valuing People: A New Strategy for Learning Disability for the Twenty-First Century (2001). London: Department of Health.

Valuing People Now: A New Three-Year Strategy for People with Learning Disabilities (2009). London: Department of Health.

S. Vehmas and P. Mäkelä (2008). 'The ontology of disability and impairment: a discussion of the natural and social features,' in K. Kristiansen, S. Vehmas and T. Shakespeare, *Arguing about Disability: Philosophical Perspectives*, 42–56. Abingdon: Routledge.

F. Vidal (1994). *Piaget Before Piaget*. Cambridge, MA: Harvard University Press.

P. Virilio (1977). *Speed and Politics: An Essay on Dromology*. New York: Semiotext(e).

M. Voysey (1975/2006). *A Constant Burden: The Reconstitution of Family Life*. Farnham: Ashgate.

E. Vul, C. Harris, P. Winkielman and H. Pashler (2009). 'Puzzlingly high correlations in fMRI studies of emotion, personality, and social cognition', *Perspectives on Psychological Science* 4, 274–290.

L. Vygotsky (1978). *Mind in Society: The Development of Higher Psychological Processes*. Cambridge, MA: Harvard University Press.

J. Walmsley, D. Atkinson and S. Rolph (1999). 'Community care and mental deficiency 1913–1945', in P. Bartlett and D. Wright (eds), *Outside the Walls of the Asylum: The History of Care in the Community 1750–2000*. London: Athlone.

M. Waltz (2008). 'Autism = death: the social and medical impact of a catastrophic medical model of autistic spectrum disorders', *Popular Narrative Media* 1(1), 13–24.

M. Waltz (2013). *Autism: A Social and Medical History*. London: Macmillan.

L. Waterhouse (2012). *Rethinking Autism: Variation and Complexity*. Amsterdam: Academic Press.

I. Watts (1811). *The Improvement of the Mind: Or, A Supplement to the Art of Logic*. London: Rivington.

F. Wesley (1989). 'Developmental Cognition before Piaget: Alfred Binet's Pioneering Experiments', *Developmental Review* 9, 58–63.

L. Wing (1975). 'Mentally retarded children in Camberwell (London)', in H. Hafner (ed.), *Estimating Needs for Mental Health Care*. Berlin: Springer.

L. Wing and J. Gould (1979). 'Severe impairments of social interaction aud associated abnormalities in children: Epidemiology and classification', *Journal of Autism and Childhood Schizophrenia* 9, 11–29.

G. Winstanley (1648). 'Truth lifting up its head among scandals', in G. Sabine (ed.), *The Works of Gerrard Winstanley*. New York: Russell and Russell.

M. Withey (2008). '"Violence", by Slavoj Žižek', *Bedeutung* 1(1), 122–127. www. bedeutung.co.uk/magazine/issues/1-nature-culture/withey-zizek-violence/. Retrieved 21 September 2014.

P. Withington (2005). *The Politics of Commonwealth: Citizens and Freemen in Early Modern England.* Cambridge: Cambridge University Press.

L. Wittgenstein (1981). *Remarks on the Foundations of Mathematics.* Oxford: Blackwell.

L. Wittgenstein (1988). *Remarks on the Philosophy of Psychology.* Chicago: University of Chicago Press.

P. Wolff and I. Meingailis (1996). 'Family patterns of developmental dyslexia: spelling disorders as behavioral phenotypes', *American Journal of Medical Genetics* 67(4), 378–386.

D. Wright (2001). *Mental Disability in Victorian England: The Earlswood Asylum.* Oxford: Clarendon Press.

R. Young (1985). *Darwin's Metaphor.* Cambridge: Cambridge University Press.

E. Young-Bruehl (2012). *Childism: Confronting Prejudice Against Children.* New Haven, CT: Yale University Press.

E. Zigler and R. Hodapp (1986). *Understanding Mental Retardation.* Cambridge: Cambridge University Press.

Index